SpringerBriefs in Reproductive Biology

W0079942

SpringerBriefs in Reproductive Biology is an exciting new series of concise publications of cutting-edge research and practical applications in Reproductive Biology. Reproductive Biology is the study of the reproductive system and sex organs. It is closely related to reproductive endocrinology and infertility. The series covers topics such as assisted reproductive technologies, fertility preservation, in vitro fertilization, reproductive hormones, and genetics, and features titles by the field's top researchers.

More information about this series at http://www.springer.com/series/11053

Alaa Hamada • Sandro C. Esteves • Ashok Agarwal

Varicocele and Male Infertility

Current Concepts, Controversies and Consensus

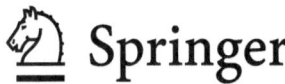 Springer

Alaa Hamada
TUFTS Medical School/St. Elizabeths
Medical Center
Boston, MA
USA

Ashok Agarwal
American Centre for Reproductive
Medicine Cleveland Clinic
Cleveland, OH
USA

Sandro C. Esteves
ANDROFERT, Andrology and Human
Reproduction Clinic
Campinas, SP
Brazil

ISSN 2194-4253   ISSN 2194-4261 (electronic)
SpringerBriefs in Reproductive Biology
ISBN 978-3-319-24934-6   ISBN 978-3-319-24936-0 (eBook)
DOI 10.1007/978-3-319-24936-0

Library of Congress Control Number: 2015957211

Springer Cham Heidelberg New York London

© The Author(s) 2016
This work is subject to copyright. All rights are reserved by the Publisher, whether the whole or part of
the material is concerned, specifically the rights of translation, reprinting, reuse of illustrations, recita-
tion, broadcasting, reproduction on microfilms or in any other physical way, and transmission or information storage and retrieval, electronic adaptation, computer software, or by similar or dissimilar
methodology now known or hereafter developed.
The use of general descriptive names, registered names, trademarks, service marks, etc. in this publication does not imply, even in the absence of a specific statement, that such names are exempt from the
relevant protective laws and regulations and therefore free for general use.
The publisher, the authors and the editors are safe to assume that the advice and information in this book
are believed to be true and accurate at the date of publication. Neither the publisher nor the authors or the
editors give a warranty, express or implied, with respect to the material contained herein or for any errors
or omissions that may have been made.

Printed on acid-free paper

Springer International Publishing is part of Springer Science+Business Media (www.springer.com)

Foreword

Varicoceles have been recognized in clinical practice for over a century. In the early years, these venous lesions were reported to have an incidence of about 16 % in the general population which is similar to the current incidence today, but the treatment of varicoceles at that time was exclusively for the management of pain. In 1952, the diagnosis and treatment of varicoceles changed dramatically. Tulloch repaired a varicocele in a man with azoospermia. Over time this man began to produce sperm in the ejaculate and he impregnated his wife. This single case report linked varicoceles and infertility, and it was soon established that the incidence of varicoceles within the infertile population was about 35–40 %. The finding of an increased incidence of varicoceles among infertile men opened a new era regarding the correction of these venous structures, but in the beginning there were only rudimentary ideas regarding many aspects of varicoceles. The pathophysiology of varicoceles was poorly understood. In addition, there was no systematic way to classify these lesions, there were no standards established to evaluate the semen parameters of these men and there were limited ways to correct these lesions. Nevertheless, most investigators agreed that varicoceles had something to do with infertility.

After 1952, innovative ideas related to varicoceles began to appear in the literature. Some of these reports included innovative corrective techniques such as micro surgery, interventional radiology, antegrade sclerosis, laparoscopy and robotic assisted varicocelectomies. Other reports on pathophysiology came from the laboratories of clinicians and reproductive scientists who studied animal models and humans with varicoceles. The early reports focused on the role increased heat that built-up within the testis and seemed to damage developing germ cells and Leydig cells. In addition, some investigators proposed that the retrograde blood flow may enable accumulation of adrenal metabolites within the testes. Over time, molecular markers and biochemical pathways were identified in men with varicoceles and these findings began to uncovered new and basic information related to the pathophysiology. For example, it was reported that the pressure effects on the walls of these varicose veins may initiate the release of Reactive Oxygen Species which have damaging effects on developing germ cells. Increased levels of germ cell apoptosis were identified in testicular histology. DNA damage was reported to be high in men with varicoceles, and this condition was reversed after a varicocele repair. In addition, the measurements of Total Antioxidant Capacity (TAC) in men with varicoceles were often low which minimized the protection of young sperm. Therefore, these findings and measurements have expanded our understanding of varicoceles and will provide the supporting evidence related to varicocele research and aspects of clinical management reported throughout this book, *Varicocele and Male Infertility*.

The authors (Alaa Hamada, M.D., Sandro C. Esteves, M.D., Ph.D., and Ashok Agarwal, Ph.D.) have written 11 chapters on different matters related to varicoceles, but each chapter is well illustrated with very educational drawings and all of the text is supported by comprehensive references that have appeared in the literature to explain the new findings related to varicocele pathophysiology. This compendium of information should be an important addition to the library of all researchers and clinicians interested in the subject of varicoceles. I have read these chapters with enthusiasm, and I intend to refer to this book over and over again.

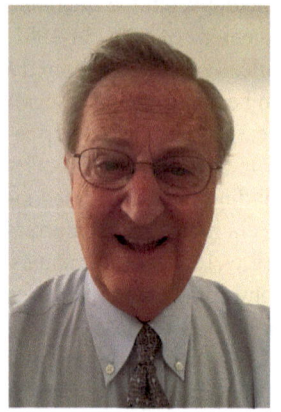

Dr. Marmar graduated from the University of Pennsylvania School of Medicine and completed his internship from Albert Einstein in Philadelphia. During internship, he met Charles Charney, M.D., who was among the first to perform varicocele surgery in the United States. Dr. Marmar was a charter member of the American Society of Andrology, Society for Male Reproduction and Urology and the Society for the Study of Male Reproduction. He was the Head-Division of Urology at Cooper Hospital for 26 years, and retired in 2013. He developed the first microsurgical varicocelectomy which continues to be used around the world. For 20 years, Dr. Marmar teamed with Susan Benoff, Ph.D., and they published many articles on the pathophysiology of varicoceles. Presently, he is the Director of Men's Health Services for Planned Parenthood of Southern New Jersey, and maintains a limited private practice for Male Infertility. Dr. Marmar is a regular reviewer for several journals and often evaluates articles related to varicoceles.

Director of Men's Health Services for   Joel Marmar, M.D.
Planned Parenthood of Southern
New Jersey

Preface

Varicocele has been one of the most controversial issues in the field of Urology and Reproductive Medicine. It is recognized as the leading cause of male infertility because it can impair spermatogenesis through several distinct pathophysiological mechanisms. Current opinion suggests that oxidative stress is the central element contributing to infertility in men with varicocele, and that surgical varicocele repair (varicocelectomy) is beneficial not only for alleviating oxidative stress-associated infertility, but also for preventing and protecting against the progressive character of varicocele and its consequent upregulations of systemic oxidative stress. Despite the advances in the understanding of this intriguing disease and consensus on some areas such as diagnosis and pathophysiology, substantial controversy still exists on the benefit of treatment and to whom treatment should be offered. With the development of intracytoplasmic sperm injection, the focus has been directed on the cost-effectiveness of interventions and patient-preferences.

Varicocele and Male Infertility: Current Concepts, Controversies and Consensus covers all the important aspects of varicocele related to infertility, from epidemiology to assisted reproduction techniques, contemplating pathophysiology, semen analysis, specialized sperm function tests, and clinical management including all available treatment options.

This authoritative article is aimed at both clinicians and scientists involved in the study and treatment of male and female fertility. This brief is intended to provide the reader with a thoughtful and comprehensive review of the clinical and scientific significance of varicocele. The text is the first of its kind, and has a broad appeal because, first it represents an invaluable tool both for basic scientists with an interest in reproductive medicine and for clinicians working in the field of infertility (e.g. urologist, gynaecologist and reproductive endocrinologist, embryologist), and second it was written in a novel in-depth manner employing evidence based medicine.

Boston, MA, USA
Campinas, SP, Brazil
Cleveland, OH, USA

Alaa Hamada, MD
Sandro C. Esteves, MD, PhD
Ashok Agarwal, PhD

Contents

About the Authors

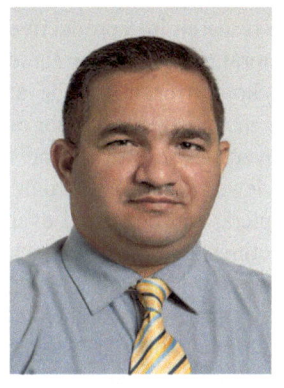

Alaa Hamada MD is currently a clinical fellow in robotic and laparoscopic urology in Tufts University and St. Elizabeth's Medical Center. Alaa Hamada is a Board-certified urologist who has done a research fellowship at Cleveland Clinic's Center for Reproductive Medicine. Since then he has completed three clinical fellowships in Robotic and Endourology in the United States (2012–2015). His clinical and research interests include male infertility, microsurgery, reproductive endocrinology and uro-oncology. Dr. Hamada has authored over 34 articles/abstracts and 8 book chapters. He is an ad-hoc reviewer of several journals such as *Urology*, *Journal of Urology* and *Andrologia*. He continues to collaborate and conduct research activities at the Cleveland Clinic, Mount Sinai Medical Center-FL and St. Elizabeth's Medical Center, MA.

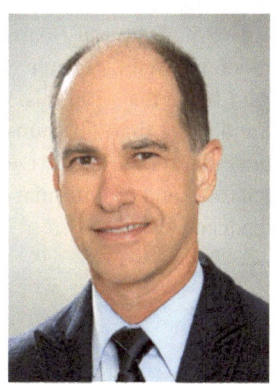

Sandro C. Esteves MD, PhD is Founder and Medical Director of Androfert, Andrology and Human Reproduction Clinic, a referral center for male reproduction in Brazil. Dr. Esteves is a Board-certified Urologist and Infertility Consultant with over 15 years of experience. Dr. Esteves received his PhD in 2001 from the Federal University of Sao Paulo, Brazil. His clinical interests include male infertility, microsurgery, reproductive endocrinology and quality management. His research interests include azoospermia-related infertility, microsurgical sperm retrieval techniques, fertility preservation, varicocele, and clean room technology. Dr. Esteves has authored over 100 scientific papers in peer-reviewed journals and more than 50 chapters in textbooks. He has co-edited journal supplements and textbooks related to infertility and IVF, including the best-selling textbook "Quality Management in ART Clinics: A Practical Guide". Dr. Esteves serves on the Editorial Board of the *Asian Journal of Andrology*, *International Urology and Nephrology, Clinics, Medical Express*, and is an Associate Editor of the *International Brazilian Journal of Urology*.

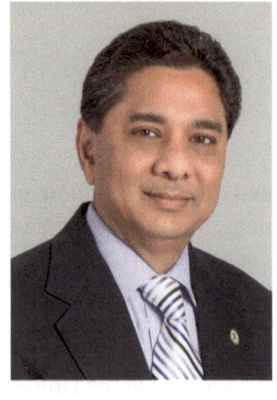

Ashok Agarwal PhD is the Director of the Andrology Center and the Director of Research at the American Center for Reproductive Medicine. He holds these positions at Cleveland Clinic, where he is a Professor at the Lerner College of Medicine of Case Western Reserve University and, since 1993, Senior Staff in Urology. Ashok did his doctorate research in reproductive biology in India and postdoctoral training in the same field at Harvard Medical School, Boston. While at Harvard, he was appointed as an Assistant Professor of Urology. He has published over 525 scientific papers and review articles in peer reviewed scientific journals, authored over 150 book chapters, and presented over 750 papers at both national and international scientific meetings. His current Hirsch index (h-index) is 93 on Google Scholar, 73 on Scopus, and 62 on Web of Science, while his citation count is 31,959 on Google Scholar. According to ResearchGate, Ashok has an RG score of 51.79 on 1494 publications. Ashok is ranked in Scopus as the #1 author in the world in the fields of Male Infertility/ Andrology and Human Assisted Reproduction, based on his number of peer reviewed publications, citation scores and h-index. He has served as an editor of over 26 medical text books/ manuals related to male infertility, ART, fertility preservation, DNA damage and antioxidants. He is the guest editor of 4 special journal issues. Ashok is a member or office bearer of several professional societies and he serves on the Editorial Board of a large number of journals in the area of reproductive medicine. Ashok is active in basic and clinical research and his laboratory has trained more than 500 basic scientists and clinical researchers from the United States and more than 50 countries. His current research interests are identifying biological markers of oxidative stress, DNA damage and apoptosis using proteomic research tools and bioinformatics analysis as well as preserving fertility in patients with cancer.

List of Figures

List of Tables

Chapter 1
Definitions and Epidemiology

Varicocele is clinically defined as a palpable elongated, dilated and tortuous testicular pampiniform plexus of veins in the spermatic cord, as shown in Fig. 1.1. It is found in approximately 15–20 % of the normal adult male population and is thought to be the most common treatable cause of male factor infertility (MFI). Its prevalence among men with primary MFI is approximately 35 % [1, 2], while 70–85 % of men with secondary infertility present with this condition [3]. In a group of 2383 patients seeking fertility care at one of the editors (SCE) tertiary center for male reproduction, varicocele was identified in 26.4 % of the individuals, as shown in Table 1.1 [4]. The high prevalence of varicocele in older males and in men with secondary MFI highlights its progressive nature [3]. On the other hand, not all men with varicocele are infertile. In fact, approximately 80 % of men with varicocele have semen parameters within the reference limits as defined by the World Health Organization reference values for semen analysis [5, 6].

Varicocele is rarely seen in the pre-adolescent age group (2–10 years), in which the estimated prevalence is about 0.92 % [7]. Large population studies, however, have shown that the prevalence of varicocele in adolescents ranges from 6 to 26 % [7–10]. In the age range of 11–19 years, varicocele was reported to affect 15 % of the subjects [8, 11, 12]. In a study involving 6200 boys aged 0–19 years, varicocele was found in 4.1 % of all the study population, whereas it affected 7.9 % of those within the age group of 10–19 years [13]. In a recent large population-based study of 1.3 million Israeli adolescent males aged 16.5–19.5 years, the prevalence of varicocele ranged from 1.6 to 4.6 % throughout the duration of the study at an average age of 17.5 years [14].

Subclinical or nonpalpable varicocele is defined by the presence of reversal of venous blood flow with Valsalva maneuver or spermatic vein ectasia with a diameter of 3 mm or greater on color Doppler ultrasonography (CDU) [15, 16]. Its estimated prevalence in the infertile population varies from 24 to 83 % [16–18]. This large variation may be due to the heterogeneity of criteria to define a varicocele on ultrasound examination. While some authors consider that the diagnosis of varicocele should be made when the vessels are larger than 3 mm, others suggest that a 2 mm cut-off for vein diameter allows for a high sensitivity of 95 % in the detection

© The Author(s) 2016
A. Hamada et al., *Varicocele and Male Infertility,* SpringerBriefs in Reproductive
Biology, DOI 10.1007/978-3-319-24936-0_1

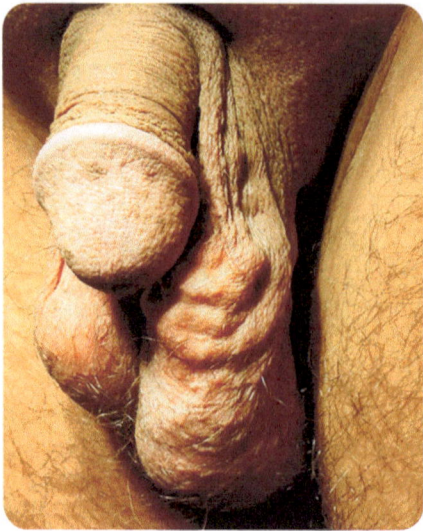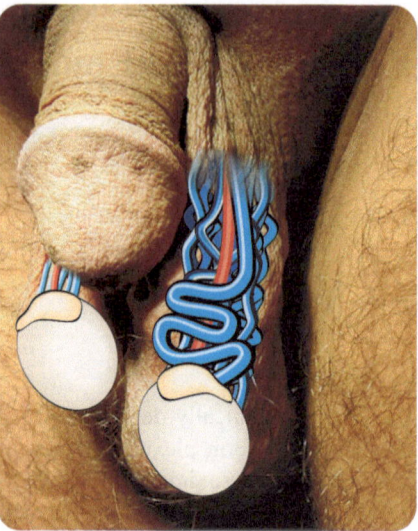

Fig. 1.1 Photograph of a large left varicocele seen through the scrotal skin (*left*). Illustration of varicose veins on the left spermatic cord as compared to normal sized-veins on the right side (*right*). (Reprint with permission from Esteves [232])

Table 1.1 Distribution of diagnostic categories in a group of infertile men attending a male infertility clinic. (Source: Androfert, Brazil; [4])

Category	N	%
Varicocele	629	26.4
Infectious	72	3.0
Hormonal	54	2.3
Ejaculatory dysfunction	28	1.2
Systemic diseases	11	0.4
Idiopathic/unexplained	289	12.1
Immunologic	54	2.3
Obstruction	359	15.1
Cancer	11	0.5
Cryptorchidism	342	14.3
Genetic	189	7.9
Testicular failure	345	14.5
Total	2383	100.0

of a varicocele [19, 20]. To complicate the matter further, it has been suggested that there is no threshold value for the ultrasonographic diagnosis of varicocele, because retrograde flow may be demonstrated in veins smaller than 2 mm in diameter [21]. As such, diagnosing a varicocele solely based on the diameter of the vessels will yield a high number of false results. As noted, such inconsistencies make it challenging to compare the results of diagnostic modalities and treatments. As far as the

CDU is concerned, it is still a matter of controversy as to which parameter is more important, namely, the reflux phenomenon or ectasia of the veins.

From a pathophysiology standpoint, varicocele has been defined as the venous incompetence that allows pathological reflux of blood to the internal spermatic vein (testicular vein) [22]. Although the treatment of varicocele has been subjected to much debate, its principle relies on the interruption of the spermatic vein continuity, thus shielding the testis from the harmful effect of venous reflux or high volume venous blood flow [23, 24].

The extent of vein structural abnormality is variable, but it usually involves dilatation of the internal spermatic veins to the level of the final drainage into the left renal vein or the inferior vena cava. Vascular dilatation may be caused by: (i) valvular incompetence of the internal spermatic veins; [25, 26] (ii) elevated hydrostatic pressure in the left renal vein, inferior vena cava, and internal spermatic veins when the patient is in the usual upright position [26]; and (iii) mechanical pressure ('nutcracker' phenomenon) from the superior mesenteric artery as it crosses the left renal vein [26].

Varicoceles are more frequently clinically detected on the left side than on the right side, and are more frequently unilateral than bilateral [18]. Based on autopsy data, it is sound to assume that the incidence of bilateral varicocele has been underestimated. Absence of valves is detected in 40 and 23 % of left and right spermatic veins, respectively, which explains the predominance of left-sided varicoceles and highlights the underestimated prevalence of right-sided varicoceles [27].

Anecdotal experience that lean men are more prone to varicocele has been supported by recent studies showing that varicocele occurrence is inversely correlated with body mass index [28, 29]. A higher prevalence in first degree relatives has also suggested an inherited pattern [30]. Also, it has been shown that long-term intense physical activity (2–4 h daily, 4–5 times a week, during 4 years) worsened semen quality in men with varicocele [31].

Key Points

- Varicocele is clinically defined as palpable elongated, dilated and tortuous testicular pampiniform plexus of veins in the spermatic cord. Subclinical or impalpable varicocele is defined based upon color Doppler ultrasound (CDU) as reversal of venous blood flow with the Valsalva maneuver or spermatic vein ectasia with a diameter of 3 mm or greater.
- Venographically, varicocele is defined as venous incompetence that allows pathological reflux into the internal spermatic vein.
- Varicocele affects 15–20 % of the normal adult male population and 35 % of men with primary male factor infertility and 70–85 % of men with secondary infertility.
- Varicocele has a progressive nature; it is rarely seen in the pre-adolescent age group and its prevalence increases progressively with age.

Chapter 2
Origin and Pathophysiology

Testicular Vein Anatomy

In this chapter, we discuss the theories attempting to explain the origin of varicocele and the pathophysiological mechanisms associated with varicocele development.

Testicular Vein Anatomy

Testicular veins emerge from mediastinum of the testis to form the pampiniform plexus, which is composed of three groups of veins, namely, the anterior, middle and posterior groups. The posterior group courses posterior to the spermatic cord and drains into the external pudendal and cremasteric veins. The latter ultimately drains into the inferior epigastric vein at the level of external inguinal ring, as shown in Fig. 2.1a. The middle group courses around the vas deferens to drain into the internal iliac vein. The anterior group courses with the internal spermatic artery. At the superficial inguinal ring, this complex form three or four tributaries that enter the pelvis. These veins eventually converge into two and then into a single internal spermatic vein running in front of the ureter and alongside the testicular artery. It is common for the main venous channel to have medial and lateral components; the lateral branch often terminates into the renal capsular, mesenteric, colonic, or retroperitoneal veins. The right internal spermatic vein enters the inferior vena cava just below the right renal vein. The left internal spermatic vein joins the undersurface of the left renal vein lateral to the vertebral column [32], as shown in Fig. 2.1b.

Variant anatomy is seen in about 20 % of cases [32, 33]. Important anomalies include drainage of the right internal spermatic vein into the right renal vein (8–10 %) and multiple terminal spermatic veins (15–20 %). Valves are present in most but not all internal spermatic veins [33].

© The Author(s) 2016
A. Hamada et al., *Varicocele and Male Infertility,* SpringerBriefs in Reproductive Biology, DOI 10.1007/978-3-319-24936-0_2

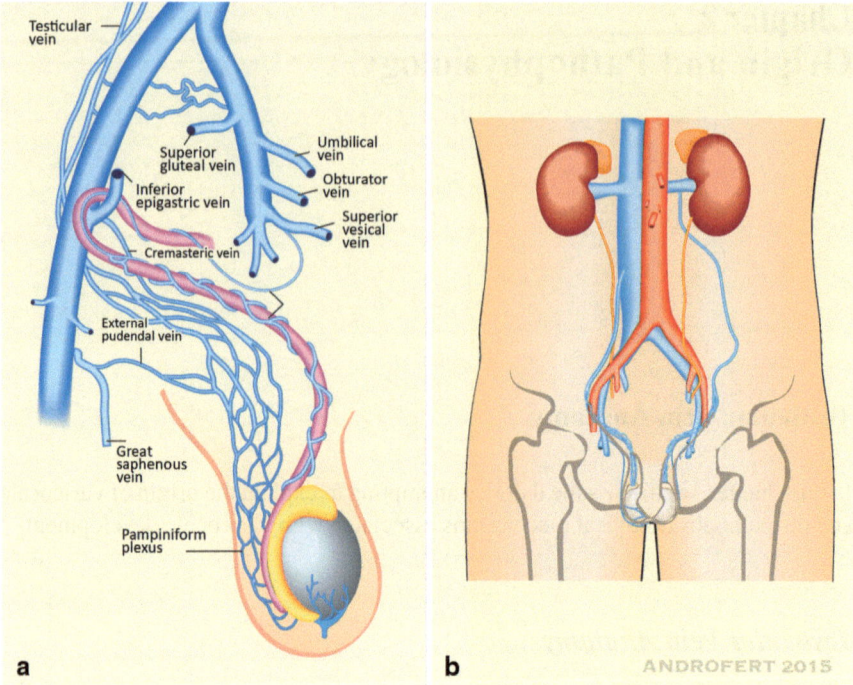

Fig. 2.1 Illustration depicting the venous testicular vasculature (**a**), and the drainage of right and left testes (**b**). The right testicular vein empties into the inferior vena cava while the left testicular vein drains into the left renal vein

Theories of Varicocele Origin

Three theories have been postulated to explain the origin of varicocele, which are not mutually exclusive. The first describes the right-angled insertion of the left testicular vein into the left renal vein, with a consequent increase in the hydrostatic pressure that is ultimately transmitted to the pampiniform plexus [26, 34]. The second relies on congenital incompetent (or absent) venous valves, resulting in retrograde flux and dilatation [18, 34]. This theory has been supported by venographic and color Doppler studies. Based upon the level of these incompetent valves being at or below the communicating veins, which include the internal spermatic, cremasteric, vassal and external pudendal veins, two pathophysiologic subtypes have been described, namely shunt and stop types, as shown in Fig. 2.2a and b. When the incompetent valves are located only above the level of the communicating veins, a stop-type varicocele is present, which constitutes 14 % of all varicoceles. The stop-type varicocele is characterized by a brief retrograde flow from the internal spermatic vein towards and into the pampiniform plexus. No orthograde venous blood flow and reflux towards the communicating veins is seen because distal valves are present and are functionally competent. Surgical ligation of the stop-type varicocele shall cure the varicocele by offsetting the reflux-producing incompetent valve

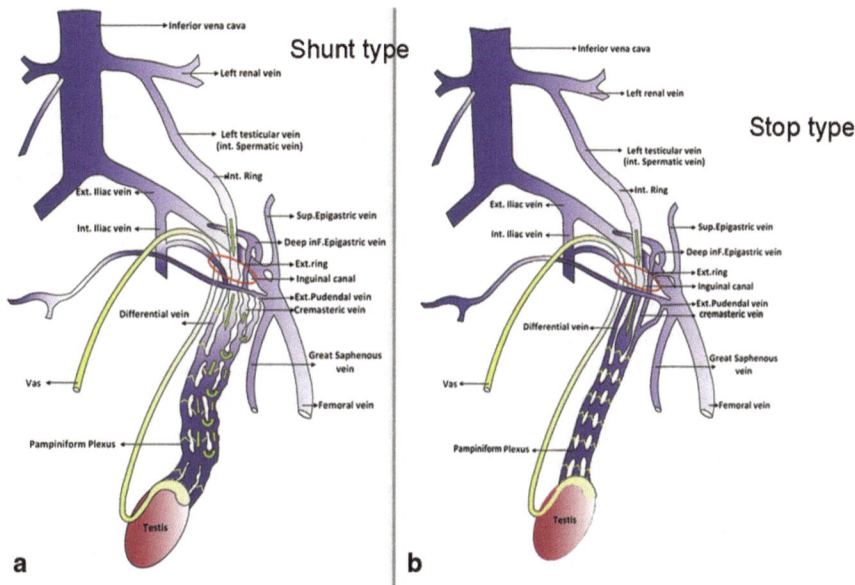

Fig. 2.2 a Schematic anatomy of the shunt-type varicocele shows incompetent valves and shunting through communicating veins, whereas in **b** stop-type varicocele, the reflux in the spermatic vein is stopped by a competent valve. (Reprinted with permission from Mohseni et al. [38])

against valves from the remaining normal venous drainage system [35]. Conversely, when incompetent venous valves are present below the communicating veins, a shunt-type varicocele is present, which constitutes 86% of all varicoceles [35, 36]. Shunt-type varicocele is characterized by retrograde blood both from the internal spermatic vein into the pampiniform plexus and orthograde reflux into the communicating veins (vasal and cremasteric veins) [37]. Surgical ligation of the shunt-type varicocele would be expected to be less effective because the incompetent valves are most numerous and widely distributed. Mohseni et al. [38] reported in a prospective controlled study involving 74 children and adolescents with varicocele that the shunt-type was associated with a greater risk of testicular hypotrophy compared to the stop-type varicocele. In addition, the authors noted that a higher recurrence rate occurred when the shunt-type varicocele had been repaired by the retroperitoneal approach compared to the inguinal approach.

The third theory involves the so-called nutcracker effect, in which compression of the left renal vein between the superior mesenteric artery and abdominal aorta would partially obstruct the blood flow through the left testicular vein and therefore increased the hydrostatic pressure inside the pampiniform plexus [39]. The nutcracker phenomenon builds up a steadily raised renocaval pressure gradient and reflux down the internal spermatic vein, resulting in the development of collateral venous pathways [40–43]. Evidence supporting this theory was provided by hemodynamic studies in adults and children with varicocele. In adults, Mali et al. [40] reported correlation between the renocaval pressure gradient and renospermatic reflux, thus showing that the severity of left renal vein compression in the upright position determines the velocity of retrograde flow in the left spermatic vein and varicocele size.

Selective left renal venography with measurement of the pressure gradient between the left renal vein (LRV) and inferior vena cava (IVC) is the gold standard diagnostic method for assessing the nutcracker effect. Normal length of the left renal vein (LRV) is 6–10 cm and the mean normal LRV diameter is 4–5 mm [7]. The normal pressure gradient between LRV and IVC is 1 mmHg or lower and an elevated gradient >3 mmHg between the LRV and the IVC can be used as a criterion of diagnosis for left renal vein entrapment [44]. Unlu et al. [45] reported using color Doppler ultrasonography that the aortomesenteric angle of men with varicocele ranged between 6–30°, which was significantly different than healthy adult males (25–50°; $p < 0.05$). Such an angle further decreases during the Valsalva maneuver in an erect position, resulting in further compression of the LRV.

Doppler ultrasonography can be used as the first diagnostic test in patients with suspected nutcracker phenomenon [43, 46]. The B-mode sonographic measurement of the diameter of the LRV combined with Doppler sonographic measurement of the peak velocity (PV) of the LRV was used to diagnose LRV entrapment syndrome. It has been suggested that the distal-to-proximal diameter ratios and flow velocity ratios exceeding 5.0 represent nutcracker phenomenon cutoff levels [43, 46, 47]. In one study involving 67 men with varicocele, 55% were demonstrated venographically to have an entrapment phenomenon [48].

The nutcracker phenomenon can be the chief cause of pediatric varicocele. In one report, children with the nutcracker phenomenon had higher grade varicocele and obvious collateral vein formation than did the patients with a lower renocaval pressure gradient [49]. However, the insufficiencies of the internal spermatic vein may be the main cause of renospermatic reflux in patients with a low renocaval pressure gradient [25, 40–42, 50, 51]. In children, the use of Doppler ultrasonography in the diagnosis of nutcracker phenomenon has been limited because the left renal vein sampling area is smaller and the Doppler angle is larger in children than in adults [47, 52].

Lastly, the etiology of varicocele may be a combination of all these mechanisms that are further aggravated by an upright posture. As shown in thin, tall athletic subjects, the incompetence of venous valves and lack of fat support around the left renal vein with narrowing of the aortomesenteric angle may lead to varicocele formation [14].

Is Varicocele a Bilateral Disease?

Historically, 85–90% of all clinical varicoceles are classified as unilateral left-sided. However, recent data indicate that bilateral palpable varicocele is found in >50% of affected men [7, 34]. Such data are in agreement with venographic studies that show bilateral abnormal venous reflux in 84–86% of men with varicocele [53–55]. This finding might explain the occurrence of bilateral testicular damage in such men, and why there is improvement in semen parameters in only 65% of men after unilateral varicocele repair [56]. In contrast, isolated right-sided varicocele is found in only 2% of patients and may be associated with the presence of an obstructive lesion, such as a retroperitoneal or pelvic compressive mass [55].

Pathophysiology

Approximately 80% of men with varicocele are fertile and have normal fecundity [5, 6]. Although the pathophysiology of varicocele has been extensively studied, no conclusive mechanism fully explains why the remaining 15–20% are infertile.

Scrotal hyperthermia, hormonal disturbances, testicular hypoperfusion and hypoxia as well as backflow of toxic metabolites are potential mediators of varicocele-mediated infertility [57]. Recently, oxidative stress has been implicated as an important mediator of varicocele-associated infertility [57]. Nonetheless, the reasons why some patients with varicocele are infertile, whereas the majority of patients are not, remain unclear. Such phenomenon may be partially explained as infertility being a combination of both male and female factors, in which a fully functional female reproductive system can compensate male factor deficiencies and therefore result in a successful conception. Different intrinsic susceptibility must exist among men with varicocele, which culminates in the various effects of varicocele on male fertility [34].

Oxidative Stress

Reactive oxygen species (ROS) are byproducts of oxygen metabolism and energy production that act as regulators of vital physiological intracellular processes. In the male reproductive tract, small quantities of ROS have important roles on sperm function—regulating capacitation, acrosome reaction, hyperactivation and the fusion of spermatozoa with the oocyte [58]. By contrast, natural intracellular and extracellular antioxidants (enzymatic and non-enzymatic) scavenge and neutralize the harmful effects stemming from increases in ROS levels. When ROS levels disproportionately increase compared with the neutralizing capacity of antioxidants, or when a reduction in the antioxidant capacity has occurred, oxidative stress usually follows.

An imbalance between ROS production and decreased total antioxidant capacity (TAC) has been implicated as the result of acidification of spermatozoa cytosol and seminal plasma in men with varicocele [59]. Oxidative stress via ROS, especially lipid peroxidation, not only damages membrane function in sperm head and midpiece altering morphology and impairing motility, but also leads to a decrease in intracellular pH. The ideal pH for ROS scavenging activity by the enzymatic antioxidant systems ranges from neutral to slightly alkaline, being markedly depressed in acidic states. Impairment of TAC may reflect as a further decrease in sperm motility [60]. These effects, however, have been speculated to vary from one subject to another according to their capacity to counteract the deleterious effects of membrane dysfunction and oxidative DNA damage. This may help understand the variable effect of varicocele on male infertility.

In a meta-analysis of studies involving oxidative stress markers in men with varicocele, we observed that oxidative stress markers were significantly increased in varicocele patients compared with normal sperm donors [60]. In one of the included studies, Mitropoulos et al. [61] evaluated oxidative stress in the peripheral blood samples of subfertile men with varicocele. The authors found an elevated level of oxidative stress due to the release of nitric oxide synthase and xanthine oxidase within the dilated spermatic vein. This led to a dramatic increase in the levels of nitric oxide, peroxynitrite, and S-nitrosothiols, all of which are biologically active. They suggested that peroxynitrite production from the reaction of nitric oxide and superoxide might be responsible for an impaired sperm function in patients with varicocele. In another study, Allamaneni et al. [62] reported that semen ROS levels correlated positively with varicocele grade. The authors showed that men with larger varicoceles had significantly higher semen ROS levels than men with small varicoceles. Similarly, Koksal et al. [63], evaluating malondialdehyde in testicular biopsy specimens, found significantly higher levels of this oxidative stress marker in infertile men with large varicoceles compared to men with small or moderate varicoceles. These findings indicate that the larger the varicocele, the higher the levels of oxidative stress. Interestingly, surgical treatment of varicocle has been shown to reduce seminal oxidative stress in such patients [64–66].

An elevated production of ROS in the reproductive tract disrupts not only the fluidity of the sperm plasma membrane, but also the integrity of DNA in the sperm nucleus. It has been shown that infertile men with varicoceles have high levels of sperm DNA damage [67]. In one study, Chen et al. [68] reported that patients with varicocele had increased levels of 8-hydroxy-2'-deoxyguanosine, a marker of oxidative DNA damage. Sperm DNA damage could also result from aberrant chromatin packaging during spermatogenesis or be a consequence of the triggering of an apoptotic-like process by ROS overproduction. Sadek et al. [69] assessed the rate of chromatin condensation using aniline-blue staining in infertile men with varicocele and showed significant improvement in DNA packing following surgical correction of large varicose veins. Excessive levels of DNA damage have been associated with a reduction in many fertility indices, including fertilization, embryo development and implantation, as well as pregnancy and live birth rates. Furthermore, DNA damage can have other significant clinical implications because *in vitro* fertilization using spermatozoa containing damaged DNA may lead to paternal transmission of defective genetic material with adverse consequences for embryonic development. Fortunately, this damage may be reversible, as shown by Zini and Libman, who recently reported that sperm DNA integrity was significantly improved in infertile men 6 months after surgical varicocele repair [70].

Recent findings reported by Blumer et al. [71] confirmed previous reports of a negative correlation between sperm morphology and the percentage of sperm with high DNA fragmentation ($r=-0.450$) in men with varicocele. Although an increase in oxidative stress as determined by the rise in malondialdehyde, which is the major product of lipid peroxidation, was not observed in the aforementioned study, a decrease in mitochondrial activity and acrosome integrity was documented. In a study involving men with palpable varicocele and oligozoospermia, Smit et al. showed significant improvement in the DNA fragmentation index (DFI) 3 months after varicocelectomy (pre-op. 35.2% ± 13.1%; post-op. 30.2% ± 14.7%, $p=0.019$) [72, 73]. A difference could also be noted between couples who conceived naturally or with assisted reproductive technology (ART) compared to those who failed (DFI%: 26.6% ± 13.7% versus 37.3% ± 13.9%, $p=0.013$). Notwithstanding, these authors demonstrated that not all patients had a decrease in sperm DNA damage after varicocele repair. In a recent work by Dada et al. [74] studying 11 men with clinical varicocele, surgical repair resulted in rapid (1 month) significant decline in free radical levels followed by slow (3–6 months) decline in DNA damage assessed by the Comet assay. On the basis of their findings, the authors of the aforementioned study recommended that infertile couples whose male partner had varicocele repair should wait 6 months after surgery before attempting to conceive. Not surprisingly, Smith et al. [72] found that high levels of sperm DNA damage were associated with varicocele even when semen analysis results were within the reference range. Of note, semen analysis as routinely performed is limited in its validity as surrogate for the assessment of male fertility potential. For this reason, it has been suggested that sperm function tests, such as sperm DNA integrity, are better indicators of male fertility potential and should be included in the semen evaluation [75, 76].

Scrotal Hyperthermia

An elevated testicular temperature has been demonstrated in men with varicocele and impaired sperm quality. Along the same lines, reduction in testicular temperature was shown to follow varicocele repair [77–81]. Because spermatogenesis is optimally at a temperature 2.5 °C lower than the core temperature, heat stress can lead to a deterioration in sperm production. However, given that most men with varicocele are fertile, and such individuals also have higher scrotal temperature than healthy men, the sole contribution of the heat stress to the infertility problem cannot entirely explain varicocele-related infertility.

The primary question is to determine whether heat stress can generate oxidative stress in the testes. Indeed, *in vitro* and *in vivo* studies have shown a direct, temperature-dependent relationship between heat exposure and generation of ROS. For instance, the exposure of *in vitro* cultures of mouse and rabbit spermatozoa to successive temperature elevation, ranging from 34 to 40 °C, but kept at constant oxygen concentrations, resulted in a concordant rise in the level of malondialdehyde [82]. Similarly, heat stress has been shown to induce increased mitochondrial, plasma membrane, cytoplasmic and peroxisomal ROS production in various human cell lines [83, 84]. Spermatogonia A, Sertoli and Leydig cells are considered thermotolerant cells as they have been previously exposed to higher temperatures in the uterus. In contrast, spermatogonia B and developing spermatozoa, particularly pachytene spermatocytes and early spermatids, are highly vulnerable to heat stress [85, 86].

Venous Hypertension and Reflux of Toxic Metabolites

Testicular venous hypertension is characterized by an excessive hydrostatic pressure column that is transmitted over the already incompetent gonadal venous valves. It is associated with a reflux of toxic adrenal and renal metabolites into the testis, including epinephrine, urea and prostaglandins E and F2α, which result in chronic vasoconstriction of testicular arterioles [87]. This phenomenon leads to persistent hypoperfusion, stasis and hypoxia, and subsequent dysfunction of the spermatogenic process [88, 89]. Microscopic evaluation of spermatic vein fragments has revealed alterations in the longitudinal muscle layers, in addition to a decrease in the number of nerve elements and "vasa vasorum" in the vessel wall. These findings suggest a defective contractile mechanism of blood transport through the pampiniform plexus. Nonetheless, a five-fold increase in hydrostatic pressure has been documented during vasography studies of the varicose spermatic veins [54], which reverses the pressure gradient and thereby lead to a hypoxic state [26, 54].

Venographic studies have shown that reversal of venous blood flow within a left-sided varicocele is common. As such, renal and adrenal metabolites can gain access to endothelial cells of the left internal spermatic vein and testicular tissue [91, 92]. These substances are known to induce cellular oxidative stress in various human cell cultures *in vitro* [93, 94]. For instance, exposure to supraphysiological levels of urea can inhibit urea transporters that mediate its cellular efflux, resulting in the carbamylation of proteins and a reduction in the level of intracellular glutathione. Carbamylation is a post-translational modification of proteins resulting from the non-enzymatic reaction between isocyanic acid and specific free functional groups. This reaction alters protein structure and therefore their functional properties. PGF-2α can induce ROS production in a variety of cell lines, whereas PGE can inhibit ROS generation. An elevated level of PGE can be attributed to endothelial cells overproduction in response to oxidative stress induced by PGF-2α. Norepinephrine can contribute to vasospasm and perpetuate hypoxia, thus aggravating ROS-mediated oxidative stress.

Apoptosis and DNA Damage

It is well known that varicocele is associated with sperm DNA damage, which has been associated with decresead fecundity [67, 95, 96]. High levels of DNA damage have also been associated with elevated ROS levels in patients with varicocele when compared with normal controls [23]. Interestingly, these differences were found in men with varicocele irrespective of impairment of semen parameters.

Varicocele is also associated with an increase in intratesticular apoptosis [89, 97]. Many apoptosis-inducing factors have been linked to varicocele-associated male infertility such as cadmium accumulation, androgen deprivation, heat stress and interleukin-6 [89, 98].

Recent Discoveries

Although an exact pathway for varicocele-induced infertility has not been completely elucidated, there is a plethora of novel studies documenting multiple derangements in the setting of varicocele. Briefly, abnormal expression of leptin receptors, glial cell-derived neurotrophic factor specific receptor GFR-*a*1 on germ cells [99, 100], and increased expression of heme oxygenase on Leydig cells are some of them [101]. In one study, Nicotina et al. [102] showed an increased expression of aquaporin receptor-1 (AQP-1) on venular endothelial cell membranes as well as Sertoli cell, diploid germ cells, and haploid cells membranes of patients with varicocele. Aquaporins are a family of transcellularmembrane proteins that mediate water transport across the cell membrane. This may indicate that in the presence of a varicocele, the testis is attempting to overcome a fluid imbalance in both tubular and interstitial compartments. In another study, Ozen et al. [103] reported a novel effect of varicocele on vas deferens motility using a rat model. The authors revealed a decline in the contractile response in the ipsilateral vas deferens compared with the contralateral vas deferens in rats with surgically-induced varicocele. Such findings suggest that other pathways, in addition to testicular damage, may take place in the presence of varicocele.

In summary, current evidence suggests that there is a multitude of mechanisms implicated in the pathophysiology of varicocele. Oxidative stress seems to be a central element contributing to infertility in such men, whose testis respond by way of, for instance, heat stress, ischemia or production of vasodilators. These responses have their own implications in exacerbating the underlying oxidative stress. The principal cells in the epididymis, the endothelial cells in the dilated pampiniform plexus and the testicular cells (developing germ cells, Leydig cells, macrophages and peritubluar cells) are the three main sites of ROS production, which include nitrogen reactive species. Varicocele-associated cell stressors induce ROS generation by distinct sperm biochemical pathways. In the mitochondria, heat and hypoxic stress can directly activate complex III of the electron transport chain to release ROS. NO, generated from testicular and endothelial cells in the testis with varicocele, can nitrosylate complexes I and IV to promote excessive release of ROS by complex III. In the sperm tail, where glycolytic units are present, NO can nitrosylate glyceraldehyde-3-phosphate dehydrogenase, contributing to intracellular acidification [59] through reducing the NADH to NAD^+ ratio and reducing the production of lactate, as shown in Figs. 2.3 and 2.4.

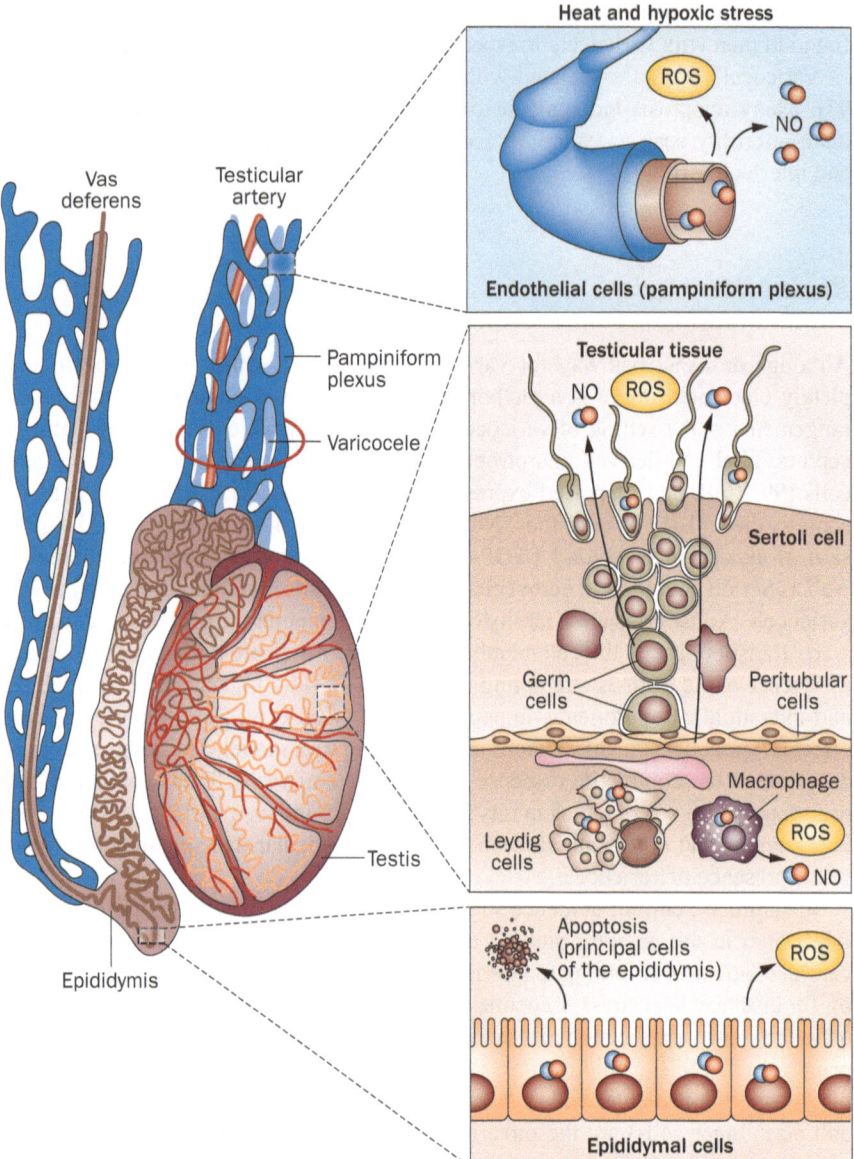

Fig. 2.3 Reactive oxygen and nitrogen species generation in infertile men with varicocele. Three components can release ROS in men with varicocele under heat and hypoxic stress: the principal cells in the epididymis, the endothelial cells in the dilated pampiniform plexus and the testicular cells (developing germ cells, Leydig cells, macrophages and peritubular cells). *ROS* reactive oxygen species

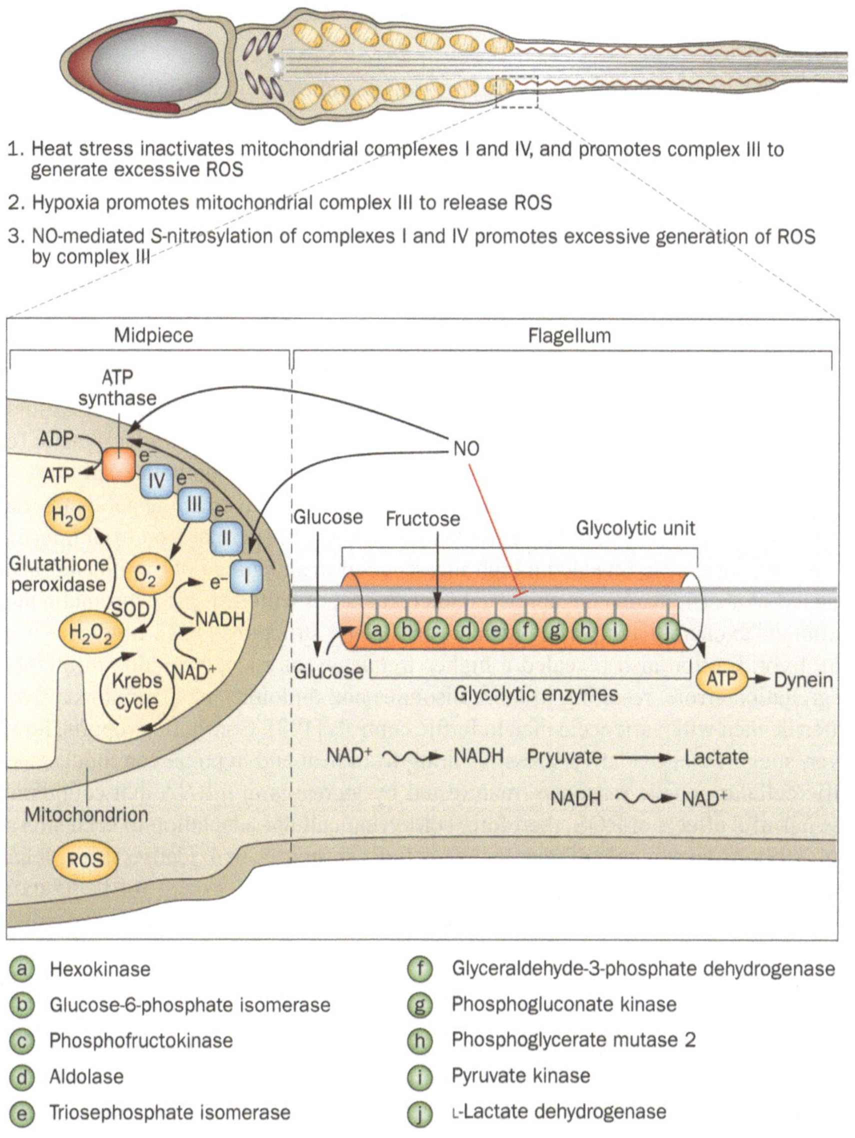

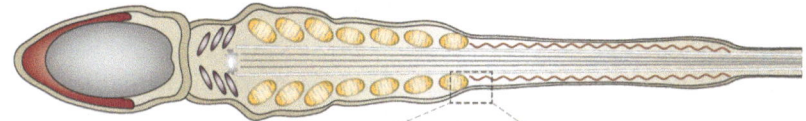

1. Heat stress inactivates mitochondrial complexes I and IV, and promotes complex III to generate excessive ROS

2. Hypoxia promotes mitochondrial complex III to release ROS

3. NO-mediated S-nitrosylation of complexes I and IV promotes excessive generation of ROS by complex III

(a)	Hexokinase	(f)	Glyceraldehyde-3-phosphate dehydrogenase
(b)	Glucose-6-phosphate isomerase	(g)	Phosphogluconate kinase
(c)	Phosphofructokinase	(h)	Phosphoglycerate mutase 2
(d)	Aldolase	(i)	Pyruvate kinase
(e)	Triosephosphate isomerase	(j)	L-Lactate dehydrogenase

Fig. 2.4 Varicocele-induced sperm biochemical pathways of ROS generation. In the mitochondria, heat and hypoxic stress can directly activate complex III of the electron transport chain to release ROS. NO, generated from testicular and endothelial cells in the testis with varicocele, can nitrosylate complexes I and IV to promote excessive release of ROS by complex III. In the sperm tail, where glycolytic units are present, NO can nitrosylate glyceraldehyde-3-phosphate dehydrogenase, contributing to intracellular acidification through reducing the NADH to NAD^+ ratio and reducing the production of lactate. *ROS* reactive oxygen species

Why Is It That Not All Men with Varicocele Are Infertile?

Although seminal markers of oxidative stress are elevated in fertile men with vari-cocele, this does not necessarily result in deterioration of fertility potential [104–106]. As aforementioned, about 80% of men with varicocele are fertile. As such, it is reasonable to speculate that certain protective mechanisms are activated to coun-teract the oxidative stress in order to protect sperm from damage. Variation in ge-netic transcriptional responses to oxidative stress might explain why most men with varicocele are fertile. Studies involving eukaryotic cells have shown that the genetic response to oxidative stress varies both among different cell lines and in response to different ROS subtypes and concentrations [107].

Unfortunately, human studies exploring the genomic and proteomic germ-cell response to oxidative stress are lacking. However, varicocele-associated cellular stressors (such as heat and hypoxia) might illicit similar and dissimilar genetic re-sponses in germ, Sertoli, Leydig, epididymal principal and endothelial cells.

Heat and hypoxia induce damage to and/or alterations in sperm genetic material and other sperm cell organelles. Electron microscopy of spermatozoa from infertile men with varicocele revealed a high incidence of disintegrated plasma membrane, reacted or absent acrosome, abnormal nuclear shapes with disrupted chromatin and deranged axonemal and periaxonemal cytoskeletal structures [108]. Fluorescent *in situ* hybridization also revealed a higher frequency of aneuploidy due to meiotic segregation errors, resulting in more disomies and diploidies in spermatozoa from infertile men with varicocele than in fertile controls [108]. Conflicting reports, how-ever, suggest that oxidative stress resulting from heat and hypoxia can induce spe-cific cellular genetic responses manifested by increases in mRNA that counteract the harmful effects of ROS, therefore, conferring cellular adaptation to such stress-ors [109]. As an example of mammalian cellular responses to oxidative stress, it has been shown that in response to exogenous H_2O_2 exposure, except for heme oxy-genase (HO), and thioredoxin reductase (TRXR), the cell antioxidant system is not inducible and is constitutive in nature [110]. With regards to varicocele, only heme oxygenase has been studied [101, 111]. Enhanced heme oxygenase expression in Leydig cells in the testes of men with varicocele is associated with the protection of these cells, maintenance of an intact testosterone milieu and process of sperm production [101]. By contrast, lower seminal levels of heme oxygenase among in-fertile men with varicocele are significantly correlated with the severity of sperm count reduction observed in these men ($p=0.001$) [111]. Currently, the mechanisms by which nuclear and/or mitochondrial genes are regulated or repressed in response to varicocele-associated cellular stressors are still unknown. We speculate that in addition to constitutively-expressed cellular antioxidants, the functional genetic re-sponse to oxidative stress is a key element for cellular survival. According to our hypothesis, germ cells can compensate for the elevated levels of oxidative stress markers measured in fertile men with varicocele, thereby protecting sperm from damage. In infertile men with varicocele, these adaptive genetic responses might be overwhelmed, culminating in sperm dysfunction and cell death.

Key Points

- No mechanism has conclusively explained infertility in men with varicocele.
- Scrotal hyperthermia, hormonal disturbances, testicular hypoperfusion and hypoxia as well as backflow of toxic metabolites are potential mediators of varicocele-mediated infertility.
- Oxidative stress has been implicated as the central mediator of varicocele-associated infertility.
- Variation in genetic transcriptional response to oxidative stress might explain why most men with varicocele retain their reproductive potential.

Chapter 3
Association Between Varicocele and Infertility

The rationale for varicocele contribution to male infertility is based on a multitude of evidence derived from epidemiologic, histologic, pre- and post-varicocele repair semen analysis and pregnancy outcomes studies.

Epidemiologic Evidence

The prevalence of palpable varicocele is higher among infertile men (21–41 %) than in the general male population (4.4–22.6 %) (112). According to the largest study on varicocele in adults ever conducted, which involved 9034 men, varicocele was found to affect 11.7 % of the total male population. Such an estimate, however, has risen to 25.4 % among the infertile male population with abnormal semen parameters (113). Furthermore, deterioration in both sperm concentration and motility was reported over time in men with varicocele [114]. The frequency of varicocele is significantly higher among men with secondary (81 %) compared to men with primary (35 %) infertility [3, 30, 115]. Such data suggests that the detrimental effect of varicocele on spermatogenesis is of a progressive nature and its testicular damaging effect is an ultimate outcome.

Evidence from Testicular Histopathology Studies

Experimental induction of left varicoceles in rats, dogs, rabbits, and monkeys resulted in deleterious effects on both testicular endocrine and exocrine function [116–118].

In humans, decrease in the ipsilateral testicular volume due to hypotrophy (arrest of ipsilateral testicular growth at time of puberty resulting in more than 10 % volume difference compared to contralateral testis) is present in approximately half of the varicocele patients [119]. In a study involving more than 4000 adolescents

© The Author(s) 2016
A. Hamada et al., *Varicocele and Male Infertility,* SpringerBriefs in Reproductive Biology, DOI 10.1007/978-3-319-24936-0_3

with varicocele, testicular hypotrophy was present in 34% of those with a grade 2 varicocele compared to 81% of those with a grade 3 varicocele, thus indicating that there is an association between varicocele size and testicular volume reduction [120]. Such reduction in testicular volume is associated with a lower total motile sperm count than that observed in varicocele patients without testicular hypotrophy [120–122].

Histologic examination of testicular biopsies of infertile men with varicocele has revealed changes in both the seminiferous tubules and interstitial tissue. A large variability in tubular diameter is observed, with a marked tubular dilatation in focal areas associated with seminiferous tubular atrophy. Variable degrees of hypospermatogenesis (germ cell hypoplasia), which denotes a decline in the number of germ cells per seminiferous tubules, is commonly seen in association with premature sloughing of immature germ cells into the lumen of the seminiferous tubules. Other histologic phenotypes include: (i) Maturation arrest, which is the failure of germ cells to proceed beyond a certain stage of spermatogenesis; (ii) Sertoli-cell-only syndrome (germinal cell aplasia), which is the complete absence of germ cells at any stage of spermatogenesis; or Sertoli cells and isolated spermatogonia; and (iii) Tubular hyalinization. Thickening of the tubular (inner) basement membranes, interstitial hyperplasia and peritubular inflammatory infiltrates are also noted [123–125].

In the lumen, in addition to sloughed cells, germ cell maturation abnormalities can be seen including spermatids with an elongated head and thin base. The Sertoli cells usually show apical cytoplasm vacuolization, dilatation of smooth endoplasmic reticulum, and alterations in the Sertoli–germ cell junctions [126]. The testicular interstitial tissue is usually swollen due to diffuse edema and an increased proliferation of collagen fibers. Dilatation of lymphatic vessels and blood stagnation in small vessels may be also observed. Leydig cells have variable appearance, namely, atrophic, hypoplastic, or hyperplasic. Surprisingly enough, Bouin's solution fixed testicular biopsies of the contralateral testis without varicocele show the same histologic alterations with slightly less severity than the ipsilateral testis with varicocele [127].

Evidence from Studies Examining Epididymis Anatomy and Function

The epididymis is a complex ductal organ, which is responsible for providing a specific intraluminal microenvironment for sperm maturation in the proximal regions and sperm storage in the distal portions. Such microenvironment is maintained both by transport between blood and lumen (and vice versa) and by synthesis and secretion of certain substances into the lumen. After passage through the epididymal duct, intraluminal hypertonicity is responsible for changes in sperm morphology to maintaining of a small volume of cytoplasmic droplet and its migration towards the sperm mid-piece [128]. Several low molecular weight organic molecules such as carnitine and inositol are present in high concentration in the epididymal lumen, but their role in sperm maturation and storage remains unclear. Metabolic processes within the epididymis are regulated by androgens [129], which are provided by both the testis via continuous free fluid transport through the efferent ducts, and the circulation.

Experimental varicocele in the animal model has been useful to study the changes in epididymal structure and function. One month after induction of varicocele in rats, reduction in epididymis weight and tubular diameter of the caput region have been observed [130]. Furthermore, terminal deoxynucleotidyl transferase dUTP nick end labelling (TUNEL) assay has shown an increased apoptosis of principal epididymal cells, which was associated with a reduction in protein and carnitine contents, as well as a decrease in α-glucosidase activity [130, 131]. Epididymal α-glucosidase activity and carnitine are markers of epididymal function and sperm content within the epididymis.

Experimental varicocele models have also shown microscopic and ultrastructural changes in the epididymal principal cells related to the duration of disease [132]. These changes include cytoplasmic vacuolation and widening of intercellular spaces. An excess of immature sperm and sperm with cytoplasmic droplets are clearly identified within the caput tubular lumen [131]. Hypoxia and heat stress are the two pathogenic mechanisms that can explain the damage and apoptosis to principal cells. Under these stressful conditions, the principal cells can overproduce ROS, which in turn causes oxidative damage to the maturing sperm and epididymal cells when combined with inadequate amount of antioxidants [133, 134].

Although human studies examining the effect of varicocele in the epididymis is scarce in the literature, certain epididymal functional markers have been examined in infertile men with varicocele. In one study, Lehtihet et al. [135] observed an increase in alpha-glucosidase, which is a specific epididymis-derived protein, from 61.7 ± 5.7 U to 84.7 ± 7.0 U ($p < 0.05$), and a decrease in sperm droplets, which is a marker of sperm immaturity, from $14.2 \pm 1.5\%$ to $11.0 \pm 1.0\%$ ($p < 0.05$), after repair of large varicoceles by embolization.

Taken together, these data indicate that reduction in fertility potential associated with varicoceles comprises both testicular and epididymal function, with a possible negative effect on sperm maturation.

Evidence from Studies Examining Conventional Semen Analysis Results

Altered semen quality is frequently seen in infertile men with varicocele. Specifically, lowered sperm counts, motility and morphology are commonplace, and these findings are often associated with tapering and amorphous spermatozoa forms [136]. Also, a high proportion of spermatozoa with alterations in the middle piece has been observed, of which the most common is residual cytoplasmic droplet [137].

Evidence from Studies Examining Specialized Sperm Function Testing

Zona Pellucida Binding

In a small study, Hauser et al. [138] examined sperm binding ability in men with varicocele-related infertility. The authors divided the patients into three groups based upon the pregnancy outcome and time to achieve pregnancy: (i) Group I consisted of three couples that achieved pregnancy within 6 months; (ii) Group II consisted of four couples who achieved pregnancy between 12–18 months; and (iii) Group III included five couples in whom pregnancy had not been recorded during the follow-up period. Sperm binding to the zone pellucida (ZP), as measured by the hemizona assay (HZA), significantly improved after varicocele repair in the groups who achieved conception, and such improvement was predictive of occurrence of pregnancy.

Sperm Penetration Assay

Vigil et al. [139], examined the sperm penetration assay by comparing three groups of men: (i) Group 1 (control) consisted of fertile men; (ii) Group 2 (experimental) consisted of infertile men without varicocele; and (iii) Group 3 consisted of infertile men with varicocele. The mean number of hamster oocytes penetrated by spermatozoa was significantly lower in infertile patients, particularly those with varicocele: $50\% \pm 8\%$ in the control, $19\% \pm 3\%$ in group 2, and $10\% \pm 3\%$ in the varicocele group ($p < 0.001$).

Hypo-Osmotic Swelling Test

The hypo-osmotic swelling test (HOST) is based on the permeability of the intact cell membrane, which causes spermatozoa to "swell" under hypo-osmotic conditions as a result of an influx of water that causes expansion of sperm tail volume. Fuse et al. [140] examined HOST in the semen of 60 men before and after varicocele repair. The authors divided the patients into two groups: (i) Group 1 consisted of 18 men with varicocele who successfully impregnated their partners, and (ii) Group 2 consisted of 42 men who did not. The authors reported that the magnitude of improvement in the HOST results after treatment was correlated with successful pregnancy outcomes.

Sperm Reactive Oxygen Species Testing

Many studies have measured seminal markers of oxidative stress in infertile men with varicocele, and compared the values obtained with those of either fertile men or infertile men with idiopathic infertility.

Malondialdehyde measurement is one of the tests that can assess oxidative stress. Malondialdehyde is a byproduct of lipid peroxidation, and can be easily measured by the thiobarbituric acid reactive substances (TBARS) assay [141]. Another method by which laboratories can test oxidative stress levels is via chemiluminescence assay. Luminol and lucigen probes can be used to determine the level of oxidative species owing to their ability to react with such molecules, upon which the probes emit a photon that can be measured using a spectrophotometer [142]. Chemiluminescence is advantageous because it can be used to measure both the intracellular and extracellular ROS levels and is, therefore, a more holistic approach to measuring oxidative species in the ejaculate than malondialdehyde measurement. Direct oxidative-stress measurements include total or specific ROS level in semen and total antioxidant capacity (TAC), whereas indirect measurements can involve the assessment of lipid peroxidation products (malondialdehyde), protein oxidation products (such as protein carbonyl) and oxidized DNA (8-hydroxy-2'-deoxyguanosine [8-OHdG]) [143]. Additionally, markers of oxidative stress have been measured in both testicular tissue biopsy specimens, and peripheral and spermatic veins blood specimens, as shown in Table 3.1A, B and C.

Controlled trials that have examined ROS levels by chemiluminescence indicate that infertile men with varicocele exhibit higher seminal ROS levels than fertile controls [62, 72, 74, 104–106, 144–147]. Higher seminal levels of specific free radicals, namely nitric oxide (NO) and nitric oxide synthase (NOS; isoform not reported), have also been detected in infertile men with varicocele compared with fertile men without varicocele [148–152]. Along the same lines, levels of hydrogen peroxide (H_2O_2) and extracellular seminal superoxide anion have been shown to be significantly higher in the semen of infertile men with varicocele than in fertile healthy controls [153, 154].

Among studies that used indirect oxidative stress assessment, the malondialdehyde assay has been the preferred method. Six out of eight controlled studies demonstrated that seminal malondialdehyde levels were significantly higher in infertile men with varicocele than in fertile healthy donors without varicocele [71, 106, 148, 152, 153, 155–157]. Other indirect markers, such as seminal hexanoyl-lysine (another lipid peroxidation product) and 8-OHdG, were also recognized to be elevated among infertile men with varicocele [149].

Direct (NO and inducible nitric oxide synthase [iNOS]) and indirect (malondialdehyde, 4-hydroxynonenal and 8-OHdG) markers of oxidative stress have been also measured from testicular biopsy specimens taken at the time of varicocele repair. In both Leydig and endothelial cells, iNOS is upregulated in infertile men with varicocele; as such, higher amounts of NO are also detected [158]. Indeed, Shiraishi et al. [159] demonstrated that large varicoceles are associated with enhanced up-

Table 3.1 Evidence of excessive oxidative stress in men with varicocele

#	Author, year and reference	OS marker	Evidence	Study group (N)	Controls (N)	Results
A. Seminal OS markers						
1.	Hendin et al. 1999 [104]	Seminal ROS (by CL)	Direct	Infertile (21) and fertile (15) men with varicocele	Sperm donors without varicocele (17)	Higher ROS levels in infertile & fertile men with varicocele
2.	Sharma et al. 1999 [145]	Seminal ROS (by CL)	Direct	Infertile men with varicocele (56)	Sperm donors (24)	Higher ROS levels in men with varicocele
3.	Pasqualotto et al. 2000 [146]	Seminal ROS (by CL)	Direct	Infertile men with varicocele (77)	Fertile men (19)	Higher ROS levels in varicocele
4.	Pasqualotto et al. 2001 [147]	Seminal ROS (by CL)	Direct	Infertile normospermic men with varicocele (16)	Healthy donors (19)	High ROS levels in varicocele group
5.	Nallella 2004 [144]	Seminal ROS levels by chemiluminescence assay	Direct	35 infertile men with varicocele	15 fertile donors	Significant elevation of ROS in semen of men with varicocele
6.	Allamaneni et al. 2004 [62]	Seminal ROS (by CL)	Direct	Infertile men with grades 2 and 3 left varicocele	Infertile men with grade 1 left varicocele	Higher ROS levels in grade 2–3 varicocele compared to grade 1
7.	Smith et al. 2006 [72]	Seminal ROS levels by chemiluminescence assay	Direct	55 with clinical varicocele, divided into normospermic and oligozoospermic	25 normozoospermic donors	ROS levels were significantly higher (P<0.01) in both groups of patients with varicocele
8.	Pasqualotto et al. 2008 [105]	Seminal ROS (by CL)	Direct	Infertile men with varicocele (21), fertile men with varicocele (15)	Fertile men (17)	Higher ROS in varicocele group
9.	Dada 2010 [74]	Seminal ROS levels by (CL)	Direct	Infertile with varicocele (11)	Healthy men (15)	Higher ROS in varicocele group
10.	Mehraban et al. 2005 [150]	Seminal NO by Griess reaction	Direct	Infertile with varicocele (40)	Infertile men without varicocele (N=40) and healthy men (40)	Significant rise in No level in semen of men with varicocele compared to other groups

Table 3.1 (continued)

#	Author, year and reference	OS marker	Evidence	Study group (N)	Controls (N)	Results
11.	Xu 2008 [151]	Seminal NO, and NO synthase (NOS)	Direct	Infertile men with varicocele (53)	Infertile men (29), fertile men (28)	Higher seminal NO level and NOS activity in men with varicocele compared to infertile men and healthy donors
12.	Sakamoto et al. 2008 [149]	Seminal NO using NO2/NO3 assay kit, 8- hydroxy-2 deoxyguanosine (8-OHdG), hexanoyl-lysine (HEL)	Direct and indirect	Oligozoospermic (15) & normozoospermic men (15) with varicocele	Normozoospermic & oligozoospermic infertile men (15) without varicocele	Higher NO, HEL 8-OHdG concentration levels in varicocele group
13.	Abd-Elmoaty 2010 [152]	Seminal MDA Colorimetric method), NO	Direct and Indirect	Infertile men with varicocele (36)	Fertile men with normal genital examination (18)	Infertile men with varicoceles showed increased levels of MDA and NO
14.	Mazzilli 1996 [154]	Extracellular seminal superoxide anion (O2-) measured by cytochrome C reduction assay	Direct	Infertile men including varicocele (132)	Fertile normozoospermic (20)	Significant increase in superoxide anion in semen of infertile men with varicocele compared to fertile men
15.	Yesilli et al. 2005 [155]	Seminal MDA	Indirect	Infertile men with varicocele (56)	Healthy men (25)	Higher seminal MDA in the varicocele group
16.	Mostafa et al. 2011 [153]	Seminal MDA, hydrogen peroxide (H₂O)	Direct and indirect	Infertile OAT men with varicocele (89)	Healthy fertile controls (20)	Grades II, III demonstrated significant increase in estimated seminal MDA, H2O2
17.	Akyol 2001 [157]	Seminal MDA (TBARS), SOD	Indirect	Varicocele patients with abnormal semen parameters (13) and varicocele patients with normal semen (12)	Healthy men (10)	No significant differences among various study groups
18.	Blumer et al. 2011 [71]	Seminal MDA	Indirect	Patients with a clinically diagnosed varicocele of grade II or III (30)	Men without varicocele (32)	No significant differences

Table 3.1 (continued)

#	Author, year and reference	OS marker	Evidence	Study group (N)	Controls (N)	Results
19.	Mostafa et al. 2009 [106]	Seminal MDA (TBARS), H_2O_2	Direct and indirect	Infertile (42) and fertile 45) men with varicocele	Fertile men without varicocele (45)	High ROS levels in varicocele groups vs. fertile men
B. Testicular biopsy						
1.	Koksal 2000 [63]	Tissue MDA levels	Indirect	15 infertile men with varicocele	10 infertile without varicocele	Higher tissue MDA levels in infertile men with varicocele and this rise is grade related
2.	Santoro et al. 2001 [158]	NO synthase (NOS) activity in testicular biopsy specimen	Direct	20 adolescents with varicocele	8 adolescents without varicocele	The iNOS is up-regulated in Leydig cells and endothelial cells in adolescents with varicocele
3.	Shiraishi et al. 2005 [101]	Generation of 4-HNE-modified proteins and Expression of Leydig cell HO-1	Indirect	30 patients with varicocele	10 healthy	Increased generation of 4-HNE-modified proteins was observed in varicocele testes and increased in Leydig cell HO-1
4.	Shirashi 2007 [159]	Intratesticular fluid NO level, testicular biopsy NOS	Direct	27 patients with varicocele	5	Increased Intratesticular level of NO and activity of iNOS in men with grade 2 and grade 3 varicocele compared to controls
5.	Ishikawa 2007 [160]	Testicular tissue 8-hydroxy-2'-deoxyguanosine (8-OHdG assessed by immunohistochemistry	Indirect	36 patients with varicocele	5	Immunostained germ cells were significantly more prevalent in the varicocele group
6.	Shirashi et al. 2009 [78]	Testicular tissue 4-HNE-modified proteins	Indirect	30 infertile men with varicocele	12 fertile men with varicocele and 10 fertile with no varicocele	Tissue 4-HNE-modified proteins was higher among infertile men with varicocele than fertile men with and without varicocele and in the left testis more than the right

Table 3.1 (continued)

#	Author, year and reference	OS marker	Evidence	Study group (N)	Controls (N)	Results
7.	Shirashi 2010 [161]	Testicular tissue 4-HNE-modified proteins	Indirect	32 infertile men with varicocele	8 healthy men	Scrotal temperature elevation is associated with higher production of 4-HNE-modified proteins
C. Spermatic veins						
1.	Mitropoulos 1996 [61]	Spermatic vein nitric oxide synthase, xanthine oxidase, nitric oxide and peroxynitrite. Serum and red blood cell antioxidant capacity was determined by a chemiluminescence reaction	Direct	5 infertile men with varicocele	No controls	Serum nitric oxide synthase and xanthine oxidase activities, as well as nitric oxide, peroxynitrite and S-nitrosothiol levels were greater in the spermatic vein compared to the peripheral vein
2.	Chen 2001 [167]	Spermatic vein plasma protein carbonyls compared to peripheral veins(spectrophotometric assay)	Indirect	30 young male patients with varicocele (group 1), 25 young male patients with subclinical varicocele (group 2)	15 normal young males without varicocele	Protein carbonyls in the spermatic veins of patients with varicocele (3.72 6 0.56 nmole/mg protein) and patients with subclinical varicocele (3.50 6 0.30 nmol/mg protein) were found to be higher than those of the control (2.35 6 0.33 nmole/mg protein)
3.	Romeo 2003 [165, 175]	Spermatic vein blood NO and peroxynitrite generation through the determination of nitrotyrosine concentration	Direct	10 adolescents with varicocele	5 controls	Plasma nitrotyrosine concentrations were significantly greater in the spermatic vein when compared with the peripheral vein
4.	Türkyilmaz 2004 [166]	Spermatic vein NO(x) (Grisse reaction) and MDA levels (TBARS) compared with the peripheral levels in the study group	Direct and indirect	13 adolescents with left varicocele of grades II–III	13 healthy children	Spermatic vein NO(x) and MDA levels were elevated significantly compared with the peripheral levels in the study group

Table 3.1 (continued)

#	Author, year and reference	OS marker	Evidence	Study group (N)	Controls (N)	Results
5.	Mostafa et al. 2006 [164]	Spermatic vein blood MDA, H2O2, NO	Direct and indirect	68 infertile men with varicococele	No controls	MDA, NO and H2O2 higher in spermatic vein than in peripheral blood
6.	Ozbek E et al. 2009 [163]	Spermatic vein blood NO using Griess reaction	Direct	20 infertile men with varicocele	15 healthy men	Significant rise in spermatic vein blood No level in of men with varicocele
Combined measurements						
1	Hurtado de Catalfo et al. 2007 [156]	TBARS (seminal and peripheral blood)	Indirect	Infertile men with varicocele (36)	Fertile men (33)	Higher ROS in infertile men with varicocele
2.	Wu Q 2009 [148]	Polymorphism in Blood glutathione S-transferase T1(GSST)and measurement of seminal Malondialdehyde (MDA), nitric oxide (NO), and total antioxidant capacity (TAC) in seminal plasma, and the mtDNA 4977 bp deletion in sperm in infertile men with varicocele	Direct and indirect	63 infertile patients with varicocele	54 healthy fertile controls	1. The frequency of the GSTT1 null genotype was 50.8% in the infertile group with varicocele and 42.6% in the control group 2. No significant relation with infertility. 3. Seminal MDA and NO is higher in infertile men with varicocele vs. controls ($P<0.05$), 4. Seminal TAC was significantly lower in the control group vs. varicocele men ($P<0.05$). 5. Infertile varicocele men with GSTT1( ) have higher OS markers than than GSTT1(+) ($P<0.05$)

CL chemiluminescence, *MDA* Malondialdehyde, *NO* Nitric oxide, *OS* Oxidative stress, *ROS* Reactive oxygen species, *TBARS* Thiobarbituric acid reactive substances regulation of iNOS. Tissue levels of malondialdehyde, 4-hydroxynonenal-modified proteins and 8-OHdG were also significantly higher in men with varicocele than in fertile healthy controls without varicocele [63, 101, 160, 161]. Koskal et al. [63, 162] observed elevated levels of malondialdehyde in human testes exhibiting severely disordered spermatogenesis, and that tissue malondialdehyde levels positively correlated with varicocele grade. The aforementioned researchers, however, failed to show a significant difference in tissue malondialdehyde levels between infertile men with varicocele and men who were infertile due to other reasons [63, 162], thus postulating that oxidative stress might be generated by different mechanisms in infertile men. In another study, Shiraishi et al. [161] showed that elevations of 4-hydroxynonenal-modified proteins in infertile men with varicocele were well-correlated with scrotal temperature elevation, but not with varicocele grade. This study supported the role of heat stress in generation of oxidative stress within testicular tissue exposed to varicocele.

Spermatic veins are essential components of the pathogenesis of varicocele-related infertility. Endothelial cells can generate excessive amounts of ROS under certain stimuli. Several studies have compared the plasma levels of iNOS, NO, xanthine dehydrogenase/oxidase, malondialdehyde, H_2O_2 and protein carbonyl content in the spermatic and peripheral veins of infertile men with varicocele as well as in controls. Plasma levels of NO and iNOS in spermatic vein of infertile men with varicocele are significantly higher than those in the peripheral blood of the same patients and healthy controls [61, 163–166]. Such findings suggest a possible contributory effect of NOS in the spermatic vein in the generation of local testicular oxidative stress. Similarly, other plasma markers, namely xanthine dehydrogenase/oxidase, malondialdehyde, H_2O_2 and protein carbonyl content, are significantly higher in the spermatic veins of infertile men with varicocele than in peripheral veins of the same patients and healthy controls [61, 164–167].

Seminal TAC, enzymatic and non-enzymatic antioxidant measurements have also been used to directly assess oxidative stress. Most controlled studies have shown that seminal TAC and specific non-enzymatic antioxidants were lower in infertile men with varicocele versus fertile healthy controls, as shown in Table 3.2 [67, 72, 105, 144–147, 168, 169]. These findings can be rationalized as non-enzymatic antioxidants, which account for approximately 65 % of the TAC, are used to scavenge excessive ROS [170].

In contrast, specific measurements of seminal antioxidant enzyme activity, particularly superoxide dismutase, which scavenges superoxide ions, have yielded conflicting results. Although the activities of seminal catalase, which detoxifies hydrogen peroxide, and glutathione peroxidase, are significantly reduced in infertile men with varicocele [106, 152, 153, 156], seminal superoxide dismutase activity can be either unchanged [157] or increased/decreased [106, 149, 152, 153, 156]. It should be noted, however, that the majority of studies assessing enzymatic antioxidants in men with varicocele have measured their specific activities rather than their concentrations. Several factors can alter antioxidant enzyme activity, such as substrate concentration (ROS levels), pH, temperature and enzyme concentration, and therefore should be adjusted to properly assess specific antioxidant enzyme activity.

Table 3.2 Evidence for decreased seminal antioxidant levels in infertile men with varicocele

#	Author, year and reference	Semen Antioxidant	Subjects (N)	Controls (N)	Results
1.	Mancini 1998 [183]	Seminal CoQ level	Infertile men with varicocele (14)	Infertile men without varicocele (23)	Oligozoospermic varicocele subjects exhibited lower cellular Co Q10 values
2.	Hendin et al. 1999 [104]	Seminal Ascorbate, urate, tocopherol & glutathione	Infertile (21) and fertile men (15) with varicocele	Sperm donors without varicocele (17)	Lower non-enzymatic antioxidants in men with varicocele vs. controls
3.	Sharma et al. 1999 [145]	Seminal TAC	Infertile men with varicocele (56)	Sperm donors (24)	Lower TAC in men with varicocele vs. controls
4.	Pasqualotto et al. 2000 [146]	Seminal TAC	Infertile men with varicocele (77)	Healthy men (19)	Lower TAC in men with varicocele vs. controls
5.	Akyol 2001 [157, 168]	Seminal SOD activity (U/ml)	Varicocele patients with abnormal spermiogram pattern (13) and varicocele patients with normal spermiogram pattern (12)	Healthy fertile men (10)	No significant differences among various study groups
6.	Pasqualotto et al. 2001 [147]	Seminal TAC	Infertile normozoospermic men with varicocele (16)	Healthy donors (19)	Lower TAC in varicocele group vs. controls
7.	Chen 2001 [167]	Seminal plasma ascorbate	Young male patients with varicocele (group 1; $N=30$); young male patients with subclinical varicocele (group 2; $N=25$)	Normal young males without varicocele (group 3; $N=15$)	Seminal plasma ascorbic acid levels in group 1 were significantly lower than those in groups 2 and 3
8.	Saleh 2003 [67]	Seminal ROS-TAC score	Infertile men with varicocele (16)	Infertile men without varicocele (15); healthy fertile controls (15)	Patients with varicoceles had significantly lower ROS-TAC scores than the infertile patients with normal genital examination or the controls
9.	Nallella 2004 [144]	Seminal TAC using a cheminescence assay	Infertile men with varicocele (35)	Fertile donors (15)	Significant reduction in TAC in semen of men with varicocele
10.	Smith 2006 [72]	Seminal TAC assessed by a chemiluminescence assay	55 with Patients with clinical varicocele, divided into normozoospermic and oligozoospermic (55)	Normozoospermic donors (25)	No significant differences

Table 3.2 (continued)

#	Author, year and reference	Semen Antioxidant	Subjects (N)	Controls (N)	Results
11.	Hurtado de Catalfo et al. 2007 [156]	Seminal Non-enzymatic antioxidants (Zn, Se), SOD activity, CAT activity	Infertile men with varicocele (36)	Fertile men (33)	Lower non-enzymatic antioxidant levels and lower enzymatic activities in infertile men with varicocele
12.	Pasqualotto et al. 2008 [105]	Seminal TAC	Infertile (21) & fertile (15) men with varicocele	Fertile men (17)	Lower TAC in varicocele groups vs. controls
13.	Mancini et al. 2007 [183]	Seminal TAC	Infertile men with varicocele (33)	varicocele (10 idiopathic oligozoo-spermic (10) and normozoospermic (24)	TAC is higher in infertile men with varicocele vs. infertile men without varicocele
14.	Sakamoto et al. 2008 [149]	Seminal SOD activity	Oligospermic (15) & Normospermic men with varicocele (15)	Oligozoospermic and normospermic infertile men (15) without varicocele	Higher SOD activity in varicocele group vs. men without varicocele
15.	Mostafa et al. 2009 [106]	Seminal SOD, catalase, GPx, vitamins C and E	Infertile (42) and fertile (45) men with varicocele	Fertile men without varicocele (45)	Lower antioxidant levels in varicocele groups vs. fertile men
16.	Giulini 2009 [168]	Seminal TAC level	Infertile men with varicocele, divided into three groups: normozoospermic (N=12), asthenozoospermic (N=8), oligo-asthenozoospermic (N=40)	10 Healthy and fertile (10)	Men with moderate oligoasthenozoo-spermia or severe oligoasthenozoosper-mia, seminal plasma TAC concentrations were significantly lower than in controls and normozoospermic patients with varicocele
17.	Abd-Elmoaty 2010 [152]	Seminal CAT, SOD, GPX, and ascorbic acid in seminal plasma	Infertile men with varicocele (36)	Fertile men with normal genital examination (18)	CAT, SOD, GPX, and ascorbic acid were significantly lower in infertile men with varicocele compared with fertile men
18.	Mostafa et al. 2011 [153]	Seminal superoxide dismutase [SOD], catalase [Cat], glutathione peroxi-dase [GPx], vit.C)	Infertile OAT men with varicocele (89)	Healthy fertile controls (20)	Decrease in seminal SOD, Cat, GPx, vit.C in varicocele-associated OAT cases when compared with the controls

Table 3.2 (continued)

#	Author, year and reference	Semen Antioxidant	Subjects (N)	Controls (N)	Results
19.	Mitropoulos 1996 [61]	Spermatic vein serum and red blood cell antioxidant capacity was determined by a chemiluminescence reaction.	5 Infertile men with varicocele (5)	No controls	Serum antioxidant capacity was greater in varicocele veins compared to peripheral veins. In contrast, the antioxidant capacity of red blood cells was less in the varicocele veins
20.	Mostafa et al. 2006 [164]	Spermatic vein blood levels of SOD, catalase glutathione peroxidase [GPx] and vitamin C)	Infertile men with varicocele (68)	No controls	Mean levels of tested antioxidants were significantly lower in the internal spermatic venous blood compared to those in the peripheral one

CAT catalase, *GPx* glutathione peroxidase, *ROS* reactive oxygen species, *SOD* superoxide dismutase, *TAC* Total antioxidant capacity

For instance, elevated scrotal temperature can result in inactivation of catalase and glutathione peroxidase because they are heat-labile enzymes [171]. The aforesaid enzymes can also undergo auto-oxidative damage by exposure to high levels of ROS [172], thus explaining their reduced activity in infertile men with varicocele despite the demonstration of heat-induced catalase gene overexpression in experimental cryptorchidism [173]. The decline in the enzymatic activities of catalase and glutathione peroxidase might explain the increase in H_2O_2 levels that has been observed in the semen of infertile men with varicocele [106, 153].

In contrast, superoxide dismutase (SOD) is a thermostable enzyme that detoxifies intracellular and extracellular superoxide anions, which results in H_2O_2 formation. H_2O_2, in turn, will ultimately be detoxified by catalase or glutathione peroxidase. Under normal conditions, intratesticular SOD levels are higher than that of catalase or glutathione peroxidase [174. Additionally, superoxide dismutase activity is generally increased in the presence of electron donors and it is inactivated in the presence of electron acceptors [175]. These features explain why SOD activity is either unchanged or increased in infertile men with varicocele [149, 157]. However, the sustained activity of SOD leads to the generation of additional testicular H_2O_2 that exceeds the detoxifying capacity of catalase or glutathione reductase, resulting in excessive oxidative stress [176]. Whether superoxide dismutase activity is inducible or constitutively expressed in infertile men with varicocele remains unclear because studies assessing the transcriptional expression of the enzyme in these men, using either mRNA determination or protein concentration, are lacking. Nevertheless, the SOD gene shows an initial increase followed by a slight decrease in response to scrotal hyperthermia [174].

Chromatin Integrity Testing

Sperm DNA fragmentation could also result from aberrant chromatin packaging during spermatogenesis or be a consequence of the triggering of an apoptotic-like process from the overproduction of ROS. Sadek et al. [69] assessed the rate of sperm chromatin condensation using aniline-blue staining in 72 infertile men with varicocele before and after repair and compared the results to 20 fertile healthy controls. The authors showed a significant decrease in the mean percentage of stained sperm heads in infertile men with varicocele (9.33 ± 13.3) 3 months following surgical correction of grade III varicose veins compared with the pre-operative levels (61.77 ± 16.8), $P = 0.043$.

Sperm chromatin integrity is reduced in men with varicocele. In a compilation of twelve studies comparing sperm DNA fragmentation (SDF) in patients with and without varicocele, SDF was significantly higher in men with varicocele (mean difference $= 9.9\%$; 95% CI: 9.2–10.5; $p < 0.0001$) [177]. In the same aforementioned study, the authors examined seven studies evaluating the effect of varicocele repair on SDF, and found that repair yielded to a significant decrease in SDF (mean difference $= 3.4\%$; 95% CI: -4.1 to -2.6; $p < 0.0001$)(177).

Evidence from Surgically-Treated Varicocele

Varicocelectomy has shown to improve at least one semen parameter, namely, sperm count, motility or morphology, in approximately 65% of the treated subjects [178]. In a meta-analysis of 17 studies that evaluated approximately 1200 infertile men with at least one abnormal semen parameter (sperm count, motility, and morphology) who had undergone high ligation or inguinal microsurgery for the treatment of palpable varicoceles, the authors showed that post-operatively, sperm count was improved by 9.7×10^6 (95% confidence interval [CI] 7.34–12.08; $P < 0.001$), sperm motility by 9.9% (95% CI 4.90–14.95; $P < 0.001$), and morphology by 3.2% (95% CI 0.72–5.60; $P = 0.01$) [179].

Regarding the influence of varicocele repair on pregnancy rates, contradictory results have been reported. In a meta-analysis by Evers and Collins [180], no benefit was verified after varicocele treatment regarding the odds of pregnancy. However, a major critique to this study was the inclusion of patients with subclinical varicocele and/or normal semen characteristics [181]. When clinically palpable varicocele coexists with impaired semen quality, current evidence supports a favorable effect of varicocele repair on pregnancy outcomes. Within this clinical scenario, Ficarra et al. [181] reviewed the randomized clinical trials for varicocele repair, and found a significant increase in the pregnancy rates for patients who underwent varicocele treatment (36.4%) compared with those having no treatment (20%) ($P = 0.009$). Similarly, Marmar et al. [182] reported a significantly higher pregnancy rates (33%) in the group of men who had undergone varicocele repair compared with those who remained untreated (15.5%; odds-ratio = 2.87; 95% CI, 1.33–6.20, $P = 0.007$). In their study, the chances of natural conception were 2.8-fold higher in the varicocelectomy group compared with the group of patients who received either no treatment or medication [182].

Key Points

- Varicocele has been associated with a reduced male fertility potential.
- Epidemiologic studies consistently reported a higher prevalence of palpable varicocele among infertile men (21–41%) than the general male population (4.4–22.6%).
- Experimental induction of varicocele in animals results in a bilateral deterioration of testicular endocrine and exocrine function.
- Animal and human studies examining the effects of varicocele on the epididymis function revealed a decrease in organ weight and a deterioration in sperm, both of which are reverted after varicocele repair.
- Histologic examination of testicular biopsies of infertile men with varicocele reveals changes in both seminiferous tubules and interstitial tissue. Predominant pathological changes include hypospermatogenesis and maturation arrest.
- Testicular growth arrest at puberty is seen in more than half of the adolescents with varicocele. Such findings are positively correlated with varicocele size.

- Altered semen quality is frequently seen in infertile men with varicocele. Stress pattern of impaired semen quality, including lowered sperm counts, motility and morphology is frequently observed, and these findings are often associated with tapering and amorphous sperm forms.
- Varicocele is associated with altered sperm function revealed by contemporary sperm function tests.
- Varicocele repair can lead to improvements in semen parameters and sperm function.

Chapter 4
Varicocele Classification

In this chapter, we examine the several classification modes have been used to diagnose and grade varicocele, including physical exam, venographic examination, color Doppler study and thermographic tests. The diagnostic accuracy of the different methods for detecting varicocele is shown in Table 4.1.

Physical Examination

Physical examination with the patient standing in a warm room is currently the preferred method for varicocele diagnosis. This method has a sensitivity and specificity of around 70 % compared with other diagnostic tools, such as venography and color Doppler studies [112, 184]. Based upon clinical examination, varicocele is generally classified according to Dubin et al. [185] into:

1. Impalpable or subclinical type or grade 0 when it is not palpable or visible at rest or during Valsalva maneuver, but demonstrable by scrotal ultrasound and color Doppler examination.
2. Palpable varicocele when it is clinically palpable at rest or with the aid of Valsalva maneuver. Such varicoceles are further divided into:
   Grade 1: Palpable only during Valsalva maneuver
   Grade 2: Palpable at rest, but not visible
   Grade 3: Visible and palpable at rest

A grade III varicocele is easily identified, as shown in Fig. 4.1, while lower grade varicoceles may be difficult to recognize particularly in certain clinical situations such as prior scrotal surgeries, cryptorchidism, obesity and hydrocele [186].

© The Author(s) 2016   37
A. Hamada et al., *Varicocele and Male Infertility,* SpringerBriefs in Reproductive
Biology, DOI 10.1007/978-3-319-24936-0_4

Table 4.1 Diagnostic accuracy of methods to detect venous reflux to the pampiniform plexus

	Sensitivity (%)	Specificity (%)	Accuracy (%)
Physical exam	70	70	67
Color Doppler ultrasound	93	85	ND
Venography	100	60–70	ND
Thermography	84–98	81–100	ND

ND not defined

Fig. 4.1 Photograph of a grade 3 varicocele

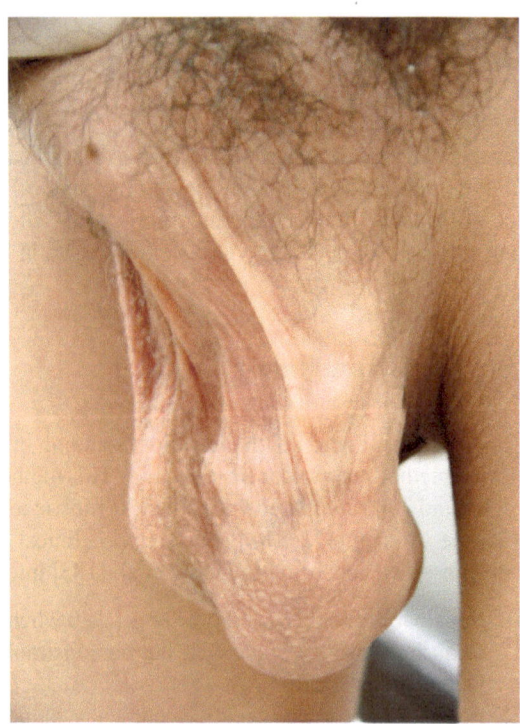

Color Doppler Ultrasonography

Whenever physical examination is inconclusive or difficult to perform as in cases of low-grade varicocele, previous scrotal surgery, obesity, concomitant hydrocele, or scrotal tenderness/hypersensitivity, imaging studies are recommended. Among the non-invasive modalities, color Doppler ultrasound (CDU) has been shown to be the best non-invasive diagnostic tool.

The ultrasound study of the scrotum should be performed with high frequency linear probes and with devices able to evaluate blood flow. Blood vessels are first studied in a grey scale and then with the color Doppler and the pulse Doppler. For the correct detection of fluxes, CDU must be calibrated to detect a slow flow (7.5 kHz). The evaluation should be performed in the supine and then the upright

Table 4.2 Scoring system for color Doppler ultrasound (CDU) diagnosis of varicocele, as proposed by Chiou et al. [188]

CDU parameter	Score
Maximum vein diameter (mm)	
<2.5-0	0
2.5–2.9	1
3.0-3.9	2
>/=4.0	3
Plexus/sum of diameter of veins	
No plexus identified	0
Plexus (+) with sum diameter<3 mm	1
Plexus (+) with sum diameter 3–5.9 mm	2
Plexus (+) with sum diameter >/=6 mm	3
Change of flow velocity on Valsalva maneuver	
<2 cm/s or duration <1 s	0
2–4.9	1
5–9.9	2

positions, with and without a Valsalva maneuver, in order to obtain a complete evaluation of the fluxes in the seminal cord veins [187].

Using the commonly accepted CDU criterion of a 3 mm or greater vein diameter for varicocele, CDU was shown to have a sensitivity of about 50% and specificity of 90% compared to physical examination [188]. It means that CDU tests negative in approximately half of the patients with palpable varicocele (low sensitivity), while it is unlikely that a patient with a non-palpable varicocele will test positive by CDU (high specificity). To circumvent this matter, Chiou et al. [188] proposed a scoring system incorporating the maximal venous diameter (score 0–3), the presence of a venous plexus and the sum of the diameters of veins in the plexus (score 0–3), and the change of flow on Valsalva maneuver (score 0–3). Using a total score of 4 or more to define the presence of CDU-positive varicocele, the authors observed a sensitivity of 93% and a specificity of 85% when compared to physical examination. In their study evaluating 64 patients, all moderate to large varicoceles found on physical examination were positive by CDU diagnosis using the scoring system, but the same group had only a 68% positive rate by traditional CDU diagnostic criteria. The scoring system for CDU diagnosis of varicocele, as proposed by Chiou et al., is shown in Table 4.2.

Pilatz et al. [189] using a 7 MHz transducer determined that the optimal vein diameter cutoff points for discriminating testicles with or without clinical varicocele was 2.45 mm in the relaxed supine position (sensitivity 84%, specificity 81%) and 2.95 mm during Valsalva maneuver (sensitivity 84%, specificity 84%).

In accordance with Sarteschi et al. [190], varicocele can be divided into five grades according to the characteristics of the reflux and its length, and to changes during Valsalva's maneuver:

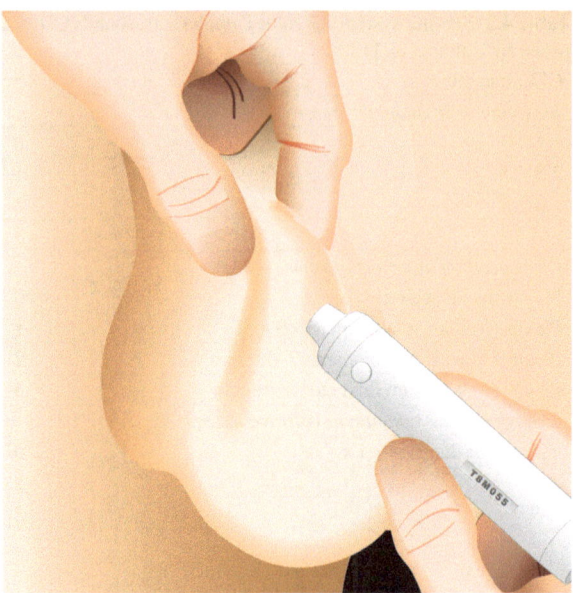

Fig. 4.2 Schematic illustration depicting the use of the 9MHz pencil-probe Doppler stethoscope for varicocele examination. The patient is examined in the upright position and the conducting gel is applied at the upper aspect of scrotum. A venous 'rush' may be heard during the Valsalva maneuver, indicating blood reflux

- Grade 1 is characterized by the detection of a prolonged reflux in vessels in the inguinal channel only during Valsalva's maneuver, while scrotal varicosity is not evident in the previous grey-scale study.
- Grade 2 is characterized by a small posterior varicosity that reaches the superior pole of the testis and whose diameter increases after Valsalva's maneuver. The CDU evaluation clearly demonstrates the presence of a venous reflux in the supratesticular region only during Valsalva's maneuver.
- Grade 3 is characterized by vessels that appear enlarged to the inferior pole of the testis when the patient is evaluated in a standing position, while no ectasia is detected if the examination is performed in a supine position. CDU demonstrates a clear reflux only under Valsalva's maneuver.
- Grade 4 is diagnosed if vessels appear enlarged, even if the patient is studied in a supine position; dilatation increases in an upright position and during Valsalva's maneuver. Enhancement of the venous reflux after Valsalva's maneuver is the criterion that allows the distinction between this grade from the previous and the next one. Hypotrophy of the testis is common at this stage.
- Grade 5 is characterized by an evident venous ectasia even in an upright position. CDU demonstrates the presence of an important basal venous reflux that does not increase after Valsalva's maneuver.

A pencil probe Doppler (9 MHz) is an inexpensive alternative to assess men with varicocele, as shown in Fig. 4.2. Examination should be carried out with the patient standing and a venous "rush" produced by blood reflux should be heard under Valsalva maneuver [4]. Although simple, this method was shown to be positive in men harboring subclinical varicocele [17]. The use of pencil probe Doppler has been advocated as an useful tool to assess subclinical varicocele on the contralateral side in a patient who already has a palpable varicocele to decide whether or not bilateral surgical repair is to be performed [191]. At present, the clinical significance of a positive result for venous reflux as shown by adjuvant diagnostic modalities such as the CDU and pencil probe Doppler in infertile men is uncertain. It is our routine, however, to examine the contralateral cord with a pencil-probe Doppler (9 MHz) stethoscope to determine if a subclinical varicocele exists when a clinically palpable varicocele is identified at one side only. Whenever present, the subclinical varicocele is treated at the same time as the coexistent clinical varicocele. This is based on the observation that altered blood flow after varicocelectomy may unmask an underlying venous anomaly and result in clinical varicocele formation [23].

Spermatic Venography

The technique of spermatic venography for varicocele diagnosis was first described by Ahlberg in 1966 [192]. It is performed using the Seldinger technique via the right femoral vein or right internal jugular vein with minor variations. Venography is often conducted in conjunction with therapeutic occlusion or in research purposes.

Briefly, the technique is performed through a transfemoral approach, the angiographer places a catheter with a single curved tip into the left or right gonadal vein to a point just beyond the valve most proximal to the left renal vein or inferior vena cava, respectively. The examiner then administers 5–10 mL of 60% iodinated contrast material by hand injection and obtains two radiographs that document the caliber of the abdominal and pelvic portions of the internal spermatic vein and show the presence of venous collateral and anastomotic channels. It is possible to look for left internal spermatic vein valvular incompetence by placing the catheter tip in the left renal vein and injecting contrast material while the patient performs a Valsalva maneuver. It is usually not necessary to image the scrotum, and gonadal shielding is both feasible and desirable.

In patients with varicoceles the internal spermatic vein diameter will be enlarged (4–12 mm), and reflux of contrast material may extend to the abdominal, pelvic, inguinal, or scrotal portions of the spermatic vein. When venography is performed in subfertile patients with palpable varicoceles, reflux is seen in nearly 100% of patients [193]. However, in subfertile patients without a palpable varicocele, left testicular reflux has been reported in 60–70% of patients [194].

Although venography is highly sensitive for detecting reflux of blood to the pampiniform plexus, its significance with reference to the presence of a clinical varicocele is unclear. Technical factors, including placement of the catheter beyond the most caudal venous valves that artificially bypasses the valves, and high injection pressure that does not reflect normal physiologic conditions are responsible for false-positives, thus lowering specificity of venographic studies [195, 196].

Marsman reported venographic findings in patients with clinical and subclinical varicoceles using nonselective and selective left spermatic vein catheterization and selective right spermatic vein cannulation [197]. A major difference between the two groups was the degree of reflux. The authors classified the degree of reflux into grades 0–5, in which grade 0 represented absence of reflux and grades 1–5 represented reflux into the upper lumbar, lower lumbar, upper pelvic, lower pelvic, or inguinal portions of the spermatic veins, respectively [197]. Sigmund and associates described two different types of varicoceles based on findings at Doppler evaluation and venography; these were the stop-type and shunt-type varicoceles [198]. In patients with stop-type varicoceles, retrograde venous reflux documented by contrast injection or by bidirectional Doppler flow signal stagnates in the internal spermatic vein. In patients with shunt-type varicoceles, retrograde venous reflux is followed by detectable increase in antegrade venous outflow through the cremasteric and deferential veins into the external pudendal, internal iliac, external iliac, and femoral veins. These authors found that in a group of 44 patients, 6 had subclinical, small, stop-type varicoceles, and 38 had clinically apparent, medium or large, shunt-type lesions [198].

Thermography

Thermography is a diagnostic method that measures temperature differences across the skin surface using non-contact telethermography utilizing infrared camera or contact thermography utilizing liquid crystals varicoscreen. Thermography was first used in medicine as early as 1957 [199], and it was applied to varicocele in the 70s. However, thermographic equipment was expensive, large in size, had poor resolution with potentially high thermal drift and there was a lack of software support for image interpretation.

Scrotal thermography was shown to be a useful diagnostic method for varicocele, because testicles have lower temperature than core body temperature in normal conditions [200]. Heat clearance by venous flow through pampiniform plexus is important to maintain this lower temperature. Given that overlaying skin temperature depends on the complex relationships of heat exchange between skin tissue, inner tissue, local vasculature and metabolic activity, venous stasis in varicocele may lead to elevated temperature of affected pampiniform plexus and/or testicle that may be detected by thermography.

Contact thermography involves the application of a flexible film containing heat-sensitive liquid crystals. This is applied to the scrotum once the patient has been undressed and upright for 5 min in a room at normal temperature. The phallus is taped to the abdominal wall to prevent interference. The thermostrips of different colors correlate with different temperatures, allowing for easy interpretation by the operator [184].

In contrast, infrared thermography allows imaging of the surface thermal distribution. Recent development of focal plane array thermovision cameras and accompanying software rendered digital thermography both less expensive and easier to standardize. The equipment consists of an E-25 digital infrared video camera (Flir Systems, Boston, MA), which has a sensitivity for temperature variance of 0.2 °C.

It is used in combination with QuickView2 software (Flir Systems) for analyzing data [201]. To perform the examination, the patients should stand in a temperature-controlled room (air temperature approximately 24 °C) with the scrotum exposed for 5 min before examination. The device records maximum and minimum temperatures of a selected area, along with average and standard deviation. The penis should be held against the abdominal wall. In healthy men the average temperature of the scrotum is symmetric and should not exceed 32 °C, corresponding to the colors blue or green. In varicocele the temperature is higher, usually between 32.5 and 35.3 °C, represented by a reddish color. Furthermore, a right–left average temperature variation of > 0.8 °C that involves more than 25 % of the hemiscrotum indicates a varicocele [202].

The discriminative value of the technique is enhanced when used in combination with the Valsalva maneuver, which further enhances the asymmetrical pattern or elevated temperature, making it particularly attractive to diagnose low-grade varicoceles. It can be also used as a follow-up method to evaluate success of varicocele treatment [202–204].

Using contact scrotal thermography, Hirsh et al. [205] reported similar accuracy for detecting varicocele compared with Doppler flow studies. Comhaire et al. [16], Lewis and Harrison [201], Kormano et al. [206], and Pochaczevsky et al. [207] have also advocated the use of scrotal thermography in evaluating patients with suspected varicoceles. However, Mieusset et al. [208] reported that increased scrotal temperatures were also observed in infertile men with abnormal spermatogenesis without varicoceles. Although scrotal thermography may also be used as an adjunctive test to confirm the clinical impression, it has not been widely employed. Further studies are needed to verify the sensitivity and specificity of non-contact thermography in diagnosis compared to CDU and venography.

Key Points

- Varicocele can be diagnosed and graded using different methods including physical examination, venography, color Doppler ultrasonography, and thermography.
- Based upon clinical examination varicocele is classified into impalpable and palpable varicocele. Palpable varicoceles are graded in: (i) Palpable only during Valsalva maneuver (grade 1); (ii) Palpable at rest, but not visible (grade 2); Visible and palpable at rest (grade 3).
- Whenever physical examination is inconclusive or difficult to perform as in cases of low-grade varicocele, previous scrotal surgery, obesity, concomitant hydrocele, or scrotal tenderness/hypersensitivity, imaging studies are recommended.
- Although venography is considered the gold standard method for diagnosing reflux of blood to the pampiniform plexus, it is rarely used except when conducted in conjunction with therapeutic occlusion.
- Among the non-invasive modalities, color Doppler ultrasound (CDU) has been considered the best diagnostic tool.
- Thermography is a diagnostic method that measures temperature differences across the skin surface using a highly sensitive non-contact telethermography utilizing infrared camera or contact thermography utilizing liquid crystals varicoscreen.

Chapter 5
Treatment Modalities

In this chapter, we discuss the therapeutic modalities that have been applied to the treatment of varicocele, including medical therapy, surgical repair and embolization technique.

Medical Therapy

Nonsurgical treatment modalities for varicocele-related infertility have been poorly studied. Use of antioxidants, anti-inflammatory and gonadotropin therapy has been attempted with conflicting results, as shown in Table 5.1.

Antioxidants and Anti-Inflammatory Agents

Oral antioxidants for varicocele-related infertility, either as a therapeutic alternative or as an adjuvant treatment to varicocele repair have been recently examined.

In a rat model of varicocele, the use of a NOS inhibitor (aminoguanidine) resulted in an increase in semen parameters and reduction in sperm DNA fragmentation [209, 210]. Vitamin E has been also shown to significantly reduce seminal ROS levels in experimental rat varicocele model [211]. In humans, daily oral administration of pentoxifylline, zinc, and folic acid for 3 months improved sperm morphology for at least 4 weeks after the end of treatment [212]. However, this evidence comes from small non-controlled series with poor methodology. In another study, Cavalleni et al. [213] studied the effects of a 6-month course of the oral antioxidants L-carnitine (1 g/day) and acetyl-L-carnitine (2 g/day) given with the anti-inflammatory cinnoxicam (30 mg suppository given every 4 days) in oligozoospermic infertile men with or without varicocele. The researchers found that both men with low-grade varicocele and idiopathic oligoasthenoteratozoospermia responded better to the combination than those who were prescribed placebo or just the antioxidants. In

© The Author(s) 2016

A. Hamada et al., *Varicocele and Male Infertility,* SpringerBriefs in Reproductive Biology, DOI 10.1007/978-3-319-24936-0_5

Table 5.1 Non-surgical modalities for treatment of infertile males with varicocele

Study	Patients	Antioxidant	Outcomes
Controlled trials			
Cavalleni et al. (2004) [213]	$n=62$ men with varicocele and 39 men with oligozoospermia treated compared with 71 men with varicocele and 47 men with oligozoospermia as controls (no treatment)	l-Carnitine (2 g/day) and acetyl-l-carnitine (1 g/day) for 6 months	Non-significant improvement in semen parameters in men with varicocele grade I and II, but significant improvement in pregnancy rate ($P < 0.01$)
Cavalleni et al. (2004) [213]	$n=62$ men with varicocele and 44 men with oligozoospermia treated compared with 71 men with varicocele and 47 men with oligozoospermia as controls (no treatment)	l-Carnitine (2 g/day), acetyll-carnitine (1 g/day) and cinnoxicam suppository (30 mg) every 4 days for 6 months	Significant improvement in semen parameters in men with varicocele grade I and II at 3 and 6 months of therapy ($P < 0.05$) and significant improvement in pregnancy rate ($P < 0.01$)
Zampieri et al. (2010) (216)	$n=73$ men with subclinical left-sided varicocele compared with 95 men with subclinical varicocele as controls (no treatment)	O-β-Hydroxyethyl-rutoside (1 g/day in a on/off 3-month cycle for 1 year)	41 % of patients in the treatment group had resolution of vein reflux within 3 years ($P < 0.05$)
Söylemez et al. (2012)(240)	$n=20$ normozoospermic men with varicocele and pain compared with 20 normozoospermic men with varicocele and pain as controls (no treatment)	Micronized purified flavonoid fraction (1 g/day for 6 months)	Relief of varicocele-associated pain in 30 % of men; improved sperm motility at 6 months ($P=0.038$) and color Doppler parameters at 1, 3 and 6 months ($P < 0.01$)
Cavallini et al. (2003) [214]	Oligozoospermic men with varicocele were divided into three groups Group 1: grade I ($n=30$), grade II ($n=4$), grade III ($n=5$) received surgery Group 2: grade I ($n=43$), grade II ($n=10$), grade III ($n=8$) received cinnoxicam Group 3: grade III ($n=40$), grade II ($n=8$), grade III ($n=6$) received placebo	Cinnoxicam suppository (30 mg every 4 days for 1 year)	Cinnoxicam significantly improved sperm quality after 2 and 4 months ($P < 0.01$) in men with grade I varicocele compared with pretreatment parameters and placebo group Cinnoxicam therapy was associated with higher sperm concentration than was seen after surgery in men with grade I varicocele, but similar improvements in sperm motility and morphology to the surgery group Stopping therapy resulted a decline to the baseline values

Table 5.1 (continued)

Paradiso Galatioto et al. [218] (2008)	$n = 20$ infertile men with persistent oligozoospermia after embolization compared with 20 infertile men with persistent oligozoospermia as controls (no treatment)	N-acetylcysteine (600 mg), vitamin C (3 mg/kg/day), vitamin E (0.2 mg/kg/day), vitamin A (0.06 IU/kg/day), thiamine (0.4 mg/kg/day), riboflavin (0.1 mg/kg/day), piridoxin (0.2 mg/kg/day), nicotinamide (1 mg/kg/day), pantothenate (0.2 mg/kg/day), biotin (0.04 mg/kg/day), cyanocobalamin (0.1 mg/kg/day), ergocalciferol (8 IU/kg/day), calcium (1 mg/kg/day), magnesium (0.35 mg/kg/day), phosphate (0.45 mg/kg/day), iron (0.2 mg/kg/day), manganese (0.01 mg/kg/day), copper (0.02 mg/kg/day) and zinc (0.01 mg/kg/day) for 90 days	Improved sperm count in 30% of men ($P = 0.009$)
Uncontrolled trials			
Kiliç et al. (2005) [217]	$n = 16$ infertile men with varicocele	Micronized purified flavonoid fraction (1 g/day for 6 months)	Relief of varicocele-associated pain in 87.5% of men; improved spermiogram and color Doppler parameters ($P < 0.001$)
Takihara et al. (1987) [219]	$n = 36$ infertile men with varicocele	Zinc sulphate (440 mg daily for 60 days to 2 years)	Significant increase in sperm motility at 2 and 12 months of therapy ($P < 0.05$)
Yan et al. (2004) (220)	$n = 30$ infertile men with varicocele	Jingling (dose NR)§	Semen parameters and pregnancy rate improved in 76.6% of men ($P < 0.01$); superoxide dismutase and zinc levels increased; cadmium levels reduced ($P < 0.01$)

a subsequent study by the same group, a 1 year course of cinnoxicam, improved the semen quality of men with low-grade varicocele [214]. Taken together, these results support the rationale of impaired fertility caused by elevated oxidative stress in men with varicocele, and the beneficial effect of improving the antioxidant defense system by exogenous antioxidant administration.

Chinese medicine exhibiting antioxidant activity has also been explored as therapeutic alternatives to surgery in animal and human studies. *Qiangjing*, a herbal medicine that was administered to rats with experimental varicocele, was found to increase glutathione peroxidase and reduce malondialdehyde in the epididymal fluid [215]. Semi-synthetic forms of bioflavonoid—a plant pigment that imparts color to flowers and displays anti-inflammatory and antioxidant properties—have also been used in men with varicocele. In one study, Zampieri et al. [216] administered 1000 mg/day of *O*-beta-hydroxyethylrutoside in a cyclical 3-month on/off therapy for 1 year to 36 infertile men with subclinical left-sided varicocele. The authors observed a slowed progression of varicocele in treated patients compared with 95 patients with subclinical varicocele who did not receive the bioflavonoid. The patients in the untreated group failed to demonstrate any protective effects against testicular growth arrest. Kiliç et al. [217] used micronized flavonoid supplements to relieve pain in normozoospermic men with varicocele and found that sperm motility was markedly improved.

Few human studies have compared antioxidant or anti-inflammatory therapy either alone of combined with surgical varicocele repair, as shown in Table 5.1. In one study, Cavallini et al. [214] showed superiority of varicocele repair in comparison with non-steroidal anti-inflammatory cinnoxicam (30 mg, suppositories used every 4 days for 12 months) to improve semen quality, especially when applied to high-grade varicoceles. In one study by Paradiso Galatioto et al. [218], the association of N-acetyl cyteine (NAC) 600 mg to a combination of vitamins and minerals (Vitamin C 3 mg/kg/day, vitamin E 0.2 mg/kg/day, vitamin A 0.06 IU/kg/day, thiamine 0.4 mg/kg/day, riboxavin 0.1 mg/kg/day, piridoxin 0.2 mg/kg/day, nicotinamide 1 mg/kg/day, pantothenate 0.2 mg/kg/day, biotin 0.04 mg/kg/day, cyanocobalamin 0.1 mg/kg/day, ergocalciferol 8 IU/kg/day, calcium 1 mg/kg/day, magnesium 0.35 mg/kg/day, phosphate 0.45 mg/kg/day, iron 0.2 mg/kg/day, manganese 0.01 mg/kg/day, copper 0.02 mg/kg/day, zinc 0.01 mg/kg/day) was able to improve sperm count in men with persistent oligozoospermia following varicocele embolization, but no effects were observed on pregnancy rates at 1-year follow-up. Contrary results were achieved by Takihara et al. [219] in a uncontrolled study with zinc sulphate therapy (440 mg for 60 days). The authors of this aforementioned study reported that not only sperm motility but also pregnancy rates were improved after varicocelectomy. Similarly, Yan et al. [220] reported increases in both seminal parameters, including reduction of oxidative stress, and pregnancy rates in 30 infertile men who received the Chinese medicine *Jingling*, which is a herbal derived substance exhibiting antioxidant effects, after surgical varicocele repair.

Despite the potential advantages of oral antioxidant/anti-inflammatory agents to varicocele patients, a definitive conclusion of its indication cannot be drawn at the present time. Most published studies have inadequate design and lack controls, which prompts an urgent need for well-designed trials. For the time being, it is sound to assume that antioxidant therapy will continue to be prescribed by urologists treating men with infertility issues with and without varicocele, despite the lack of firm evidence supporting its routine prescription [221].

Surgical Treatment

The principle of surgical treatment is the interruption of the spermatic vein continuity, thus shielding the testis from the harmful effect of venous reflux or high volume venous blood flow, and therefore restore or improve testicular function.

Patient Selection

Current recommendations suggest that treatment should be offered for couples with documented infertility whose male partner has a clinically palpable varicocele and abnormal semen analysis. Given the diagnosis of such condition is mainly clinical, a detailed medical history and physical examination must be taken, and prognostic factors identified. Physical examination with the patient standing in a warm room is the preferred diagnostic method, as discussed in Chap. 4. When physical examination is either inconclusive or equivocal, such as in cases of low-grade varicocele and in men with a history of previous scrotal surgery, concomitant hydrocele or obesity, imaging studies may be recommended [184, 222].

Pre-operative workup should include hormone profile testing particularly, follicle stimulating hormone (FSH) and testosterone level. Testicular volume should be assessed using a measurement instrument such as the Prader orchidometer or a pachymeter [4]. At least two semen analyses must be obtained and evaluated according to the World Health Organization guidelines [223].

Infertile men undergoing varicocele repair for large varicoceles are more likely to show—semen parameters improvement [224]. On the other hand, reduced pre-operative testicular volume, elevated serum FSH levels, diminished testosterone concentrations and subclinical varicocele are negative predictors for fertility improvement after surgery [89, 203, 225–229].

Men with clinical varicoceles presenting with azoospermia may be candidates for surgical repair. In such cases, genetic evaluation including Giemsa karyotyping and polymerase chain Yq microdeletion screening for AZFa, AZFb and AZFc regions are recommended. A testis biopsy (open or percutaneous) may be obtained to assess testicular histology, which has been shown to be the only valid prognostic factor for restoration of spermatogenesis [230, 231]. The benefit of varicocelectomy in azoospermic men with genetic abnormalities is doubtful and should be carefully balanced. The same caution is valid for patients with atrophic testes and/or history of cryptorchidism, testicular trauma, orchitis, systemic or hormonal dysfunction because varicocele in such cases may not be the cause of infertility but merely coincidental.

As for all restorative surgical procedures in male infertility, the evaluation of the female partner's reproductive potential is recommended before an intervention is indicated, and the alternatives to varicocele repair fully disclosed.

Surgical Techniques

The aim of surgical treatment of varicocele to infertile men is to offer the highest improvement in the male fertility status with low complication rates. Because the estimation of natural pregnancy after treatment is difficult to ascertain due to a variety of factors, including the lack of a uniform post-treatment follow-up interval and female factor parameters such as age and reproductive health, the ultimate treatment goal is to improve the male fertility potential regardless of the method to be used for conception (unassisted or assisted). The ideal surgical technique should aim for ligation of all internal and external spermatic and cremasteric veins, with preservation of spermatic arteries and lymphatics.

Anesthesia

Anesthesia for varicocelectomy may be carried out using local, regional or general type, according solely with the surgeon and patient's preferences. It is our preference to perform microsurgical subinguinal varicocele repair using short-acting propofol intravenous anesthesia associated with the blockage of the spermatic cord using 10 mL of a 2 % lidocaine hydrochloride in an outpatient basis [230, 232].

Techniques

Both open (with or without magnification) and laparoscopic approaches are the surgical methods for varicocele treatment. The high retroperitoneal and laparoscopic approaches are performed for internal spermatic vein ligation while the inguinal and subinguinal approaches allow the ligation of the internal and external spermatic and cremasteric veins that may contribute to the varicocele [34, 232].

Open Retroperitoneal High open retroperitoneal varicocele ligation involves incision medial to the anterior superior iliac spine at the level of the internal inguinal ring, as shown in Fig. 5.1. The external oblique muscle is split, the internal oblique muscle is retracted and the peritoneum is teased away. Exposure of the internal spermatic artery and vein is carried out retroperitoneally near the ureter. At this level, only one or two internal spermatic veins are seen, but the internal spermatic artery may not be easy to identify. The veins are ligated near to the point of drainage into the left renal vein. As shown in Fig. 2.1a, neither the parallel inguinal and retro-

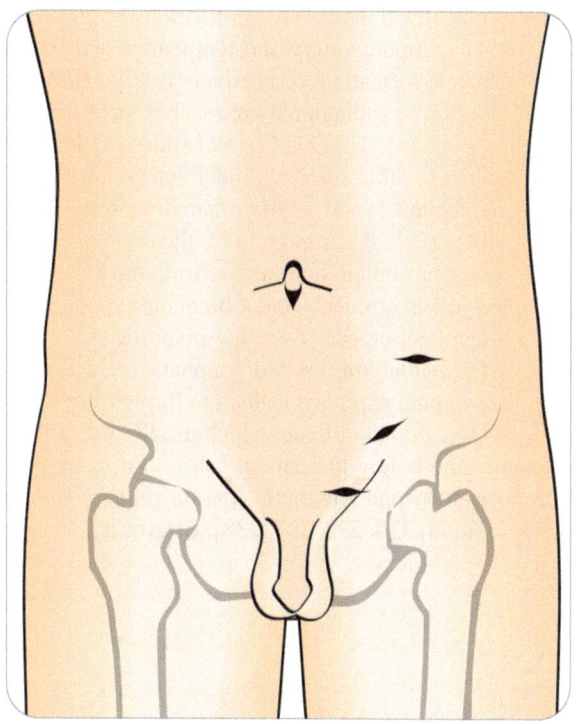

Fig. 5.1 Incision sites used for subinguinal, inguinal and retroperitoneal open surgical varicocele repair. In the subinguinal approach, a transverse incision is made just below the level of the external inguinal ring. An oblique incision is made along the axis between the anterior superior iliac spine and the pubic tubercle for the inguinal approach. In the retroperitoneal approach, a transverse incision is made medial to the anterior superior iliac spine. (Reprint with permission from Esteves [232])

peritoneal collateral veins that exit the testis and bypass the retroperitoneal area of ligation nor the cremasteric vein can be identified in the retroperitoneal approach. It is believed that these collaterals cause recurrence of varicocele, as noted by the high recurrence rate after retroperitoneal open varicocele ligation. The surgical approach on the right side may be more difficult because the right testicular vein drains in the inferior vena cava, as shown in Fig. 2.1b.

Laparoscopic Laparoscopic varicocelectomy is essentially a retroperitoneal approach using high magnification. The spermatic artery and the lymphatics are easily identified and spared. The collateral veins can also be clipped or coagulated. However, the external pudendal vein, a common cause of varicocele recurrence, is not accessible (see Fig. 2.1a). This shortcoming of laparoscopic varicocelectomy leads to a recurrence rate of approximately 5 % [233]. Laparoscopy varicocele repair is more invasive, costly and it is associated with higher complication rates than open procedures [233–235].

Inguinal and Subinguinal The classic approach in inguinal varicocelectomy involves an incision over the inguinal canal, opening of the external oblique aponeurosis and isolation of the spermatic cord, as shown in Fig. 5.1. The internal spermatic veins are dissected and ligated. An attempt is made to identify and spare the testicular artery and lymphatics. The external spermatic veins running parallel to the spermatic cord or perforating the floor of the inguinal canal are identified and ligated. Although the internal and external spermatic veins can be identified

macroscopically, the use of magnification facilitates identification and preservation
of internal spermatic artery and lymphatics, which may prevent testicular atrophy
and hydrocele formation, respectively [236]. Microsurgical varicocelectomy either
using inguinal or subinguinal approaches has been considered the best method for
varicocele repair [34, 232, 237]. Nevertheless, these procedures requires more skill
as compared to other surgical modalities because a higher number of internal spermatic vein channels and smaller-diameter arteries are seen at the level of the inguinal canal. As such, it is important for the urologist who opts to treat varicocele using
microsurgery to obtain appropriate training. It is also important to have adequate
microsurgical instruments and a binocular operating microscope with foot-control
zoom magnification because loupe-magnification is insufficient for proper identification of testicular arteries and lymphatics. The main advantage of the subinguinal
over the inguinal approach is that the former obviates the need to open the aponeurosis of the external oblique, which usually results in more postoperative pain and
a longer time before the patient can return to work. Our preferred method is the
testicular artery and lymphatic-sparing subinguinal microsurgical repair, as shown
in Fig. 5.2 [34, 230, 232, 237, 238]. Briefly, a 2.5 cm skin incision is made over the

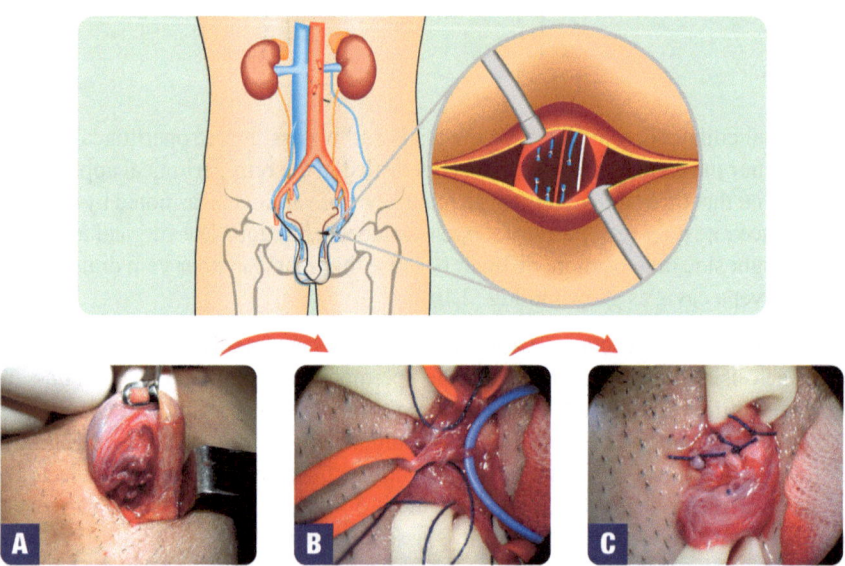

Fig. 5.2 Illustration depicting a left subinguinal microsurgical varicocelectomy. A 2 cm transver-
sal skin incision is made immediately below the external inguinal ring. The muscle layers and the
inguinal canal are not violated. The spermatic cord is exteriorized and the cremasteric veins are
identified and ligated (**a**). In panel B, the spermatic cord was dissected to allow the identification
of the testicular artery (*blue* vessilloop), dilated varicose veins (*red* vessilloops), and lymphatics (*blue* cotton sutures). While testicular artery and lymphatic channels are preserved, dilated
veins are ligated with non-absorbable sutures and transected (**c**). (Adapted with permission
from Esteves and Miyaoka R. Surgical Treatment for Male Infertility. In: Parekattil SJ, Agarwal
A (Eds). Male Infertility: Contemporary Clinical Approaches, Andrology, ART & Antioxidants.
Springer, New York, 1st ed. 2012, pp. 55–78)

external inguinal ring. The subcutaneous tissue is separated until the spermatic cord is exposed. The cord is elevated with a Babcock clamp and the posterior cremasteric veins are ligated and transected. A Penrose drain is placed behind the cord without tension. The cremasteric fascia is then opened to expose the cord structures and the dissection proceeds using the operating microscope with magnification ranging from 6 to 16×. Dilated cremasteric veins within the fascia are ligated and transected. Lymphatics and arteries are visually identified and preserved. Whenever needed, the cord structures are sprayed with papaverine hydrochloride to increase the arterial beat and ease identification of testicular arteries. Alternatively, an intraoperative vascular Doppler flow detector can be used to identify and spare arteries [239]. All dilated veins of the spermatic cord are identified, tagged with vessel loops, then ligated using non-absorbable sutures and transected. Vasal veins are ligated only if they exceed 2 mm in diameter. Sclerosis of small veins is not used.

Postoperative Follow-Up

Postoperative care usually includes local dressing and scrotal supporter for 48–72 h and 1 week, respectively. Scrotal ice packing is always recommended to control local edema for the first 48 postoperative hours. Patients are counseled to restrain from physical activity and sexual intercourse for 2–3 weeks. Oral analgesics usually suffice to control postoperative pain. Postoperative follow-up aims to evaluate improvement in semen parameters, complications and pregnancy outcome. Semen analysis should be performed every 3 months until the semen parameters stabilize or pregnancy occurs.

Results of surgical varicocele repair. In a recent systematic review comparing different surgical modalities to treat varicocele for male infertility [233], it was concluded that open microsurgical inguinal or subinguinal varicocelectomy techniques resulted in higher rate of natural pregnancy and fewer recurrences and postoperative complications than laparoscopic, radiologic embolization and macroscopic inguinal or retroperitoneal varicocelectomy techniques, as shown in Table 5.2. Hydrocele formation is the most common complication of varicocelectomy, with the incidence ranging from 0 to 10 %. The lowest and highest reported hydrocele formation rates are seen with the microsurgical and high retroperitoneal methods, respectively. Recurrence rates, which range from 0 to 35 %, are also technique-dependent. Acciden-

Table 5.2 Comparison of post-operative recurrence, hydrocele formation and natural pregnancy rates among the surgical modalities for treatment of infertile males with varicocele

Technique	Recurrence (%)	Hydrocele formation (%)	Natural pregnancy (%)
Open retroperitoneal	7–35	6–10	25–55
Laparoscopic	2–7	0–9	14–42
Macroscopic inguinal	0–37	7	34–39
Microscopic (inguinal or subinguinal)	0–0.3	0–1.6	33–56

Values are expressed as a range

tal testicular artery ligation during microsurgical varicocelectomy has been reported to be about 1 %, and it may cause testicular atrophy. It has been recently demonstrated that use of intraoperative vascular Doppler during microsurgical varicocelectomy allowed more arterial branches to be preserved and more internal spermatic veins to be ligated [239].

Key Points

- Medical therapy, including antioxidants and anti-inflammatory agents have been utilized to treat symptomatic men with varicocele and infertility in men with varicocele with variable success. A definitive conclusion of its indication cannot be drawn at the present time because most published studies have inadequate design and lack controls.
- Varicoceles are surgically treated either by open (with or without magnification) or laparoscopic approaches. The principle of the surgery is the occlusion of the dilated veins of the pampiniform plexus. The high retroperitoneal and laparoscopic approaches are performed for internal spermatic vein ligation while the inguinal and subinguinal approaches allow the ligation of the internal and external spermatic and cremasteric veins that may contribute to the varicocele.
- Open microsurgical inguinal or subinguinal varicocelectomy techniques result in higher rate of natural pregnancy and fewer recurrences and postoperative complications than laparoscopic, radiologic embolization and macroscopic inguinal or retroperitoneal varicocelectomy techniques.
- The aim of surgical treatment of varicocele in infertility is to offer a chance to completely or partially restore the male fertility status with lower complication rates. The ultimate treatment goal is to increase the likelihood of establishing a pregnancy irrespective of the method of conception, i.e., natural or assisted.

Chapter 6
Subclinical Varicocele

Subclinical varicocele refers to the presence of varicose veins in the pampiniform plexus that are not palpable during physical examination, but are detected by adjunctive diagnostic tools, including Doppler examination, color Doppler ultrasound, scrotal thermography and venography [17, 112, 184, 188, 189, 222].

Evidence supporting treatment of infertile men with subclinical varicocele is equivocal [203, 241–243]. Only two randomized controlled trials have examined the efficacy of varicocele repair in men with subclinical varicocele. In one study, Unal et al.[244] randomized a total of 42 infertile men with left subclinical varicocele to surgery and medical therapy with 50 mg/day of clomiphene citrate. The authors observed a significant improvement in sperm density and motility in the surgery compared with the medication group, but no differences in pregnancy outcomes were reported. Yammamoto et al randomized 85 infertile me with subclinical varicocele diagnosed with thermography. Likewise the study of Unal et al., an improvement in the sperm density and motility was observed, but no differences in pregnancy rates were noted (203).

Notwithstanding, the management of infertile men with a clinical varicocele at one side and a subclinical one at the contralateral side has been debated. The question is whether or not bilateral varicocele ligation should be offered to such patients. In an attempt to solve this dilemma, Zheng et al. [245] compared the efficacy of bilateral and left unilateral varicocelectomy in a group of 104 infertile men with left clinical and right subclinical varicoceles. The authors of this aforementioned study found that bilateral varicocelectomy had no significant advantage over the left clinical varicocelectomy. In their study, however, a retroperitoneal approach was used for vein ligation, which was shown to be associated with high recurrence rate [233]. Contrary results have been achieved by Elbendary and Elbadry [246], who performed a prospective study involving 145 men with the same characteristics as mentioned in the study of Zheng et al. In their study, however, varicocelectomy was performed using an inguinal open technique. Although a significant improvement in sperm parameters was observed in both groups, the magnitude of change in sperm count and motility, as well as natural pregnancy rates, was significantly higher in the group of men who had bilateral varicocele repair, as shown in Table 6.1. Their find-

© The Author(s) 2016   55
A. Hamada et al., *Varicocele and Male Infertility,* SpringerBriefs in Reproductive Biology, DOI 10.1007/978-3-319-24936-0_6

Table 6.1 Summary of studies examining semen parameters and pregnancy outcomes in infertile men with subclinical varicocele

Studies	Patients no	Design	Therapy	Diagnostic method	Outcomes
Unal 2001 [244]	42 infertile men with subclinical varicocele	RCT	Group 1: ($n=21$) Clomiphene citrate Group 2 ($n=21$) Varicocele repair	CDU	Sperm density and motility significantly improve in group 2 only. PR: in group $1=12.5\%$ and in group $2=6.7\%$ with no statistical significance ($p=0.5$)
Pasqualotto 2005 [250]	50 infertile men with varicocele	Prospective controlled	Group I ($n=30$): Left-sided grades 2 and 3 varicoceles and absence of contralateral subclinical varicocele; Group II ($n=20$): Left-sided grades 2 and III and right subclinical varicocele	CDU	Mean sperm concentration in Group II increased significantly ($30.32 +/- 9.8$; $p=0.03$). Pregnancy rate was higher in Group II (66.7%) compared to Group I (33.3%)
Yamamoto et al. 1996 [203]	85 infertile men with subclinical varicocele	RCT	Group I ($n=45$): Varicocelectomy Group II ($n=40$): Observation	Infrared thermography	Improved sperm density and motility in group I. PR: 6.7% in group I compared to 10% in group 2 ($p>0.05$)
Dhabuwala et al. 1996 [23]	54 infertile men	Retrospective	Group 1 ($n=38$): palpable varicocele treated with surgery Group 2 ($n=16$): subclinical varicocele treated with surgery	CDU	Spermiograms improved in 76% of the patients in group 1 and in 81% of the patients in group 2. Similar pregnancy rates in groups 1 (47%) and 2 (50%)

ings are in agreement with early studies suggesting that bilateral varicocelectomy is more effective than unilateral repair to such patients [23, 247]. The rationale of bilateral varicocelectomy when a concomitant clinical and subclinical varicoceles are found relies on the hypothesis that there might be an alteration in blood flow following unilateral clinical varicocelectomy which may unmask an underlying contralateral venous anomaly resulting in a clinically manifested varicocele [247].

Noteworthy, current clinical guidelines do not support the repair of subclinical varicoceles as an attempt to overcome infertility [243, 248, 249]. Nevertheless, given the scarceness of well-designed studies there is a need of more investigation to determine whether any subset of patients with subclinical varicocele and infertility could benefit from intervention.

Key Points

- Subclinical varicocele refers to presence of impalpable varicocele that has been detected with adjuvant methods such as color Doppler ultrasound, scrotal thermography and venography.
- At present, there is no firm evidence supporting the therapeutic role of varicocele repair in infertile men with subclinical varicocele.
  Some authors have advocated the concomitant repair of subclinical varicocele contralateral to the clinical varicocele, based on the assumption that one-sided repair may lead to altered fluid hemodynamics and progression of subclinical variocele.

Chapter 7
Varicocele in Adolescents

Adolescent varicocele have been associated with testicular volume loss, endocrine abnormalities, and abnormal semen parameters [251]. Severe testicular damage is found in 20 % of adolescents affected, with abnormal findings in 46 % of affected adolescents. Histological findings are similar in children or adolescents and in infertile men. In 70 % of patients with grade 2 and 3 varicocele, left testicular volume loss was found.

In about 20 % of adolescents with varicocele, fertility problems will arise [113]. Improvement in sperm parameters has been demonstrated after adolescent varicocelectomy [252–254]. Therefore, varicocele repair has been recommended to adolescents presenting palpable varicocele and ipsilateral testicular growth retardation greater than 2 mL or two standard deviations from the mean of the normal testicular growth curve. Those presenting with normal ipsilateral testicular volume, however, should be offered follow-up monitoring with annual measurement of testicular size or semen analyses because varicocele can progress [243]. Nevertheless, due to the complexity to evaluate testicular growth retardation in adolescents presenting with bilateral varicocele or solitary testis, varicocelectomy should be considered in such cases.

Although testicular hypotrophy is the most widely accepted indication for repairing adolescent varicocele, it should be noted that testicular size may not be a reliable indicator of fertility potential in patients with varicocele [253]. Therefore, semen analysis may be discussed with older adolescents in an effort to facilitate the decision of whether or not to treat the varicocele. In cases of abnormal seminal parameters associated with high-grade varicocele, the consensus is that surgery should be offered, even when testicular size is normal.

Notwithstanding, the literature is scarce in studies determining what are the reference ranges for semen analysis results in this population, presumably because of ethical concerns associated with the procurement of semen specimens in young boys [252, 254]. In a study involving adolescents (14–18 years of age) attending a public school in Brazil, it was determined whether the grade of varicocele influenced semen quality and testicular volume [255]. Sperm progressive motility and concentration were significantly lower in adolescents with grades 2 and 3 varicocele

© The Author(s) 2016
A. Hamada et al., *Varicocele and Male Infertility,* SpringerBriefs in Reproductive Biology, DOI 10.1007/978-3-319-24936-0_7

compared with adolescents without varicocele, but the magnitude of change was not different according to varicocele grade. The total number of progressively motile sperm in the ejaculate was also lower in varicocele grades 2 and 3, and adolescents with varicocele grade 3 presented lower number of progressively motile sperm compared with those with grade 2. Interestingly, despite having markedly lower semen analysis results than the counterparts without varicocele, the adolescents with varicocele still had their semen parameters within the World Health Organization reference ranges, thus indicating that conventional parameters such as count, motility and morphology may not accurately discriminate those in which varicocele already affect fertility and who might benefit from intervention [34, 256]. In the aforementioned study by Mori et al. [255], testicular asymmetry was significantly less prevalent in adolescents without varicocele. Among the adolescents, 27.8 % (95 % confidence interval [CI]: 23.2, 32.4) presented varicocele grades 2 and 3. There was a high prevalence of testicular asymmetry in adolescents with left grade 2 (41.7 %) and 3 varicocele (51.9 %), whereas only 11 % of the adolescents without varicocele showed minimal testicular asymmetry.

As far as the effect of varicocele repair in adolescents is concerned, the consensus is that treatment may be effective, but caution should be exercised to not overtreat these subjects [257]. Several authors reported on reversal of testicular growth after varicocelectomy in adolescents. Kass and Belman [258], in a study involving 20 adolescents aged 11–19 years with grades 2 and 3 varicocele and ipsilateral testis hypotrophy, showed that varicocelectomy led to a significant catch-up growth of the treated testis. In this study, all patients were followed for 1–6 years. The authors' data indicated that a moderate to large varicocele was responsible for testicular growth retardation, and early ligation of the varicocele may revert this process. These findings have been corroborated by others, indicating that among adolescents with pre-operative left hypotrophy who underwent varicocelectomy, about 70 % achieve catch-up growth within 28 months follow-up [259, 260]. The average proportion of catch-up growth of 76.4 % (range: 52.6–93.8 %) has been found according to a recent meta-analysis [261].

While some have suggested laparoscopic and subinguinal microscopic varicocelectomies as an alternative to reduce the incidence of hydroceles, which is more common after Palomo and Ivanissevich repair, the optimal choice for the operative approach in the treatment of adolescent varicocele continues to be debated [262]. Some form of optical magnification (microscopic or laparoscopic) has been advocated because the internal spermatic artery is 0.5 mm in diameter at the level of the internal ring and it allows lymphatic-sparing varicocelectomy to be performed [263, 264]. The recurrence rate with ligation methods involving optical magnification is usually <10 %, and they aid preventing hydrocele formation, thus helping testicular hypertrophy development and better testicular function according to the LHRH stimulation test [236, 264, 265].

Key Points

- Adolescent varicoceles may be associated with testicular volume loss, endocrine abnormalities, and abnormal semen parameters.
- Moderate and large varicocele can be responsible for testicular growth retardation and that early ligation of the varicocele can reverse this process.
- Varicocele repair has been recommended to adolescents who have palpable varicocele and ipsilateral testicular growth retardation greater than 2 mL or two standard deviations from the mean of the normal testicular growth curve.
- To adolescents with palpable varicocele who have normal ipsilateral testicular volume, the consensus is to follow-up monitoring with annual measurement of testicular size and semen analyses (if appropriate) because varicocele can progress.
- While some have suggested laparoscopic and subinguinal microscopic varicocelectomies as an alternative to reduce the incidence of hydroceles, which is more common after Palomo and Ivanissevich repair, there is no consensus on the optimal choice for the operative approach.

Chapter 8
Effect of Varicocele Treatment

Although multiple pathophysiological derangements have been documented in varicocele, the central issue is whether or not repair of this condition improves fertility. Much debate has centered on this question, and rightfully so, as it is the bottom-line for both clinicians and patients. In this chapter, we examine the impact of varicocele treatment on male fertility parameters such as semen parameters, specialized sperm function tests and natural as well as assisted pregnancy rates.

Impact on Semen Parameters

Varicocelectomy studies report significant im in one or more semen parameters in approximately 65 % of the treated men [56]. In a recent meta-analysis, Agarwal et al. [179] combined 17 observational studies and randomized controlled trials using sophisticated methods to minimize selection bias as described by the Potsdam Consultation [266]. Overall, sperm concentration, motility and morphology were increased by 9.7 million/mL, 10 and 3 %, respectively, after varicocelectomy. The mean amount of time for semen improvement and natural pregnancy after surgery was approximately 5 and 7 months, respectively [179, 267].

The reasons the why fertility potential is not always improved in varicocelectomized patients are still obscure, and robust data is lacking to determine prognostic factors that might help identify the best candidates for treatment. From the limited available data, it seems that infertile men undergoing surgery for large varicoceles are more likely to benefit from varicocelectomy [56, 267, 268]. As far as age is concerned, an interesting report suggested that advanced paternal age does not influence the fertility outcomes of men with varicocele-associated infertility. It should be noted, however, that results might be biased by the fact that the group of men older than 40 years had a significantly higher proportion of subjects with secondary infertility as opposed to the other study with younger individuals [269].

© The Author(s) 2016
A. Hamada et al., *Varicocele and Male Infertility,* SpringerBriefs in Reproductive Biology, DOI 10.1007/978-3-319-24936-0_8

Impact on Sperm Function

Oxidative Stress

It is believed that oxidative stress (OS) represents the central pathogenic mechanism for testicular damage in men with varicocele-related infertility. Several studies have been conducted examining resolution of markers of oxidative stress in these patients. Varicocelectomy has been shown to decrease or normalize the common 4977-bp mitochondrial DNA deletion [270], 8-OHdG [159, 270], TBARS [64, 156], and nitrate plus nitrite content [149], all of which are OS markers elevated in spermatozoa of infertile men with varicocele. Additionally, varicocele repair has been shown to improve or normalize the levels of seminal and peripheral blood plasma total antioxidant capacity (TAC) [65, 156] as well as seminal antioxidants such as alpha-tocopherol [64, 156], ascorbate [64, 156, 270], retinol [156], selenium [156], and zinc [156]. Several studies have also demonstrated that varicocele repair can reduce total and specific markers of seminal reactive oxygen species (ROS) elevation (malondialdehyde, H_2O_2, nitric oxide, 8-OHdG and hexanoyl-lysine) [64, 74, 149, 156, 270]. However, one controlled [155] and two uncontrolled [240, 271] studies failed to show any beneficial effect of varicocele repair on the alleviation of oxidative stress (Table 8.1). In a study by Yeşilli et al. [155], lactate dehydrogenase (LDH), LDH-X activities, and lipid peroxidation product (malondialdehyde [MDA]) levels were unchanged after varicocelectomy. However, the authors of this aforementioned study showed that sperm HspA2 activity, which is a biochemical marker of sperm maturity, was increased postoperatively compared with pre-operative values ($p < 0.001$).

Along the same lines, Rodriguez Peña et al. [271] failed to observed changes in nitric oxide concentrations after varicocele repair . Their study, however, included varicocele patients with no history of infertility that might have biased their results. Lacerda et al. [272] showed that varicocele repair was associated with no demonstrable beneficial effect of varicocelectomy in reducing seminal levels of malondialdehyde in adolescents with varicocele, despite a positive effect on sperm DNA integrity and mitochondrial activity. The aforesaid authors speculated that varicocele repair was unable to alter the levels of seminal plasma oxidative stress because these levels were not elevated pre-operatively in their group of adolescents, and suggested that varicocele itself does not alter seminal plasma lipid peroxidation in this particular subset of patients. However, it is still unknown whether a time-dependent effect of varicocele on markers of OS will occur in adolescents at later age.

Some studies have also examined blood levels of thiobarbituric acid reactive substances (TBARS) and plasma peroxidation susceptibility lag time (a marker of antioxidant levels) in spermatic veins and peripheral veins before and after varicocele repair. A marked reduction in peripheral vein plasma TBARS levels, indicating a decrease in ROS, and a significant increase in plasma peroxidation susceptibility lag time, indicating an increase in the antioxidant levels, have been observed several months to 1 year after repair, as shown in Table 8.1 [65, 156].

Table 8.1 Effects of varicocele repair on oxidative stress markers in infertile men

Study	Patients	Postoperative markers of oxidative stress	Postoperative antioxidants	Conclusions
Mostafa et al. (2001) [64]	$n=68$ men undergoing varicocelectomy	At 3 and 6 months, seminal malondialdehyde (both $P=0.0001$), H2O2 (both $P=0.0001$) and NO ($P=0.0002$ and $P=0.00014$, respectively) were reduced	At 3 and 6 months, superoxide dismutase (both $P=0.0001$) catalase (both $P=0.0001$), glutathione peroxidase (both $P=0.0001$), vitamin C (both $P=0.0001$) were increased and vitamin E (both $P=0.0001$) were reduced albumin levels were increased at 6 months ($P=0.0001$) but not at 3 months ($P=0.2$)	Varicocelectomy reduces seminal oxidative stress
Yes, illi et al. (2005) [155]	$n=56$ with 25 healthy controls	At 6 months, no change in seminal malondialdehyde levels ($P=0.65$); sperm HSPA2 activities increased significantly compared with preoperative levels ($P<0.001$)	NR	Varicocelectomy does not reduce oxidative stress but positively impacts sperm maturation
Cervellione et al. (2006) [65]	$n=11$	At 1 year, reduced plasma TBARS assay ($P=0.003$)	At 1 year, increased plasma peroxidation susceptibility lag time ($P=0.0025$)	Varicocelectomy reduces peripheral blood oxidative stress
Hurtado de Catalfo et al. (2007) [156]	$n=36$ with 33 fertile controls	At 1–3 months, reduced seminal and peripheral TBARS assay ($P 0.001$) After 3 months, reduced seminal NOS levels ($P 0.001$), but peripheral blood levels were unchanged At 1 month, seminal protein carbonyl levels have normalized	Reduced preoperative seminal zinc and selenium levels normalized 3 months after surgery; reduced preoperative seminal total antioxidant capacity normalized 6 months after surgery; reduced preoperative ratio of seminal glutathione to oxidized glutathione normalized 6 months after surgery; reduced preoperative intracellular sperm content of vitamin C, α-tocopherol and retinol levels normalized 3–6 months after surgery; increased preoperative sperm content of glutathione reductase, glutathione peroxidase and glutathione transferase normalized 1 month after surgery; elevated preoperative peripheral blood erythrocyte, spermatic vein erythrocytes and sperm levels of superoxide dismutase and catalase normalized 8 months after surgery	Varicocelectomy reduces oxidative stress

Table 8.1 (continued)

Study	Patients	Postoperative markers of oxidative stress	Postoperative antioxidants	Conclusions
Chen et al. (2008) [283]	$n = 30*$	At 6 months, reduced seminal 8-OHdG ($P < 0.001$)	At 6 months, seminal protein thiol and ascorbate levels increased ($P < 0.001$)	Varicocelectomy reduces oxidative stress
Sakamoto et al. (2008) [149]	$n = 15$ oligozoospermic men with varicocele undergoing varicocelectomy	At 6 months, reduced seminal 8-OHdG (0.001), NO (0.001) and hexanoyl-lysine ($P < 0.005$)	At 6 months, high preoperative superoxide dismutase levels normalized	Varicocelectomy reduces oxidative stress
Rodriguez Peña et al. (2009) [271]	$n = 202$	At 6 months, no change in seminal NO levels	NR	Varicocelectomy does not reduce oxidative stress in men with no history of subfertility
Dada et al. (2010) [74]	$n = 11$ with 15 fertile controls	At 1 and 3 months, reduced seminal ROS levels ($P < 0.001$)	NR	Varicocelectomy reduces oxidative stress
Lacerda et al. (2011) [272]	$n = 27$ adolescents (15–19 years) with grades II or III varicocele	At 3 months, no difference in seminal malondialdehyde levels	NR	Varicocelectomy does not reduce oxidative stress in adolescents

By contrast, the clinical interpretation of studies assessing seminal antioxidant response to varicocele repair poses a more complex problem. For non-enzymatic antioxidants, such as vitamin C, retinol, zinc, selenium, protein thiols and albumin, most studies have shown pre-operative reduced levels and significant postoperative increases to normal levels [64, 74, 149, 156, 270]. With regards to vitamin E, although one study showed that low pre-operative levels can be normalized postoperatively, [156] a contrary report demonstrated a significant reduction in vitamin E levels 3–6 months after varicocelectomy [64]. However, since vitamin E is an essential vitamin and its levels in body fluids are influenced by dietary intake, no definite predictive value for its measurement in semen can be anticipated to reflect the balance between oxidants and antioxidants without controlling for the diet. As far as the activities of enzymatic antioxidants are concerned, two studies demonstrated that seminal superoxide dismutase (SOD), and intracellular superoxide dismutase, catalase (CAT) and glutathione peroxidase (GPx) activities were elevated in men with varicocele, all of which were reduced after surgery [149, 156]. In contrast, Mostafa et al. [64] observed a significant increase in post-operative seminal plasma levels of SOD, CAT, GPx.

Although some observations suggest that seminal enzymatic antioxidants exhibit lower activities in infertile men with varicocele than fertile men, which might be attributed to auto-oxidation as well as protein unfolding and degradation. Additional studies are needed to resolve the discrepancy in the results as shown by different researchers.

Notably, the time required to observe any improvement in oxidative stress markers after varicocele repair is variable. In one report, Dada et al. [74] showed that decline in ROS levels after varicocelectomy was proportional to the length of the postoperative period. In their study, damage to sperm DNA, which usually takes extended periods to revert to normal status, improved only after 6 months. Mostafa et al. [64] observed that markers of seminal oxidative stress (NO, H_2O_2 and malondialdehyde) were significantly reduced whereas antioxidant levels of superoxide dismutase, catalase, glutathione peroxidase and vitamin C were elevated 3 and 6 months after varicocele repair. In another report, Hurtado de Catalfo et al. [156] showed that levels of non-enzymatic antioxidants (zinc and selenium) and the proportion of sperm exhibiting DNA fragmentation were still abnormal 1 month after varicocele repair, while levels of reduced and oxidized seminal glutathione and antioxidant enzymes were normalized as compared with age-matched fertile controls. Additionally, Chen et al. [270] demonstrated that sperm mitochondrial DNA deletions and 8-OHdG were reduced whereas seminal plasma protein thiols and ascorbic acid levels were elevated 6 months after varicocele repair compared with their preoperative levels. Lastly, Sakamoto et al. [149] found that a time lag of approximately 6 months is required to achieve a marked improvement in seminal ROS markers, such as NO, 8-OHdG and hexanoyl-lysine, after varicocele repair.

The importance of measuring oxidative stress in varicocele and the observation of oxidative stress alleviation after varicocele repair stems from two interesting findings. First, these markers might help to predict the response of varicocele repair in infertile men. Accordingly, Shiraishi et al. [66], analyzing levels of testicular

4-hydroxynonenal-modified proteins before varicocelectomy, found that men who responded to varicocelectomy by increasing postoperative sperm count, motility and morphology had higher basal levels of preoperative testicular modified proteins than non-responders ($p = 0.014$). More importantly, the researchers recognized that varicocelectomy was not as effective in men without oxidative stress, thus supporting the rationale that patients with high levels of OS should be considered the ideal candidates for varicocelectomy [66]. Second, some reports indicate that there is a relationship between resolution of the markers of oxidative stress and improvement in semen parameters and sperm quality postoperatively [64, 156]. For instance, Hurtado de Catalfo et al. [156] observed improvements 3 months after surgery in both semen parameters (sperm concentration and morphology) and blood testosterone levels, which were concomitant to improvements in seminal zinc, selenium, protein carbonyl and DNA fragmentation levels. Along the same lines, Mostafa et al. [64] observed significant improvements in sperm count, motility and morphology, in accordance to improvements in seminal levels of malondialdehyde, H_2O_2, NO, superoxide dismutase, catalase, glutathione peroxidase and vitamin C, 3 and 6 months after varicocele repair, as shown in Table 8.1 [64]

In summary, current evidence demonstrates that varicocele repair can alleviate oxidative stress and normalize antioxidant defense systems, and, therefore, aid in restoring or improving fertility. Furthermore, data suggest that this beneficial effect is time-dependent, with greater results being achieved 6 months after surgery. Oxidative stress biomarkers may be useful to monitor postoperative outcomes after varicocele repair. Ideal candidates for varicocele repair seem to be subjects with palpable varicocele who present with abnormal semen parameters or sperm function tests, including oxidative stress.

Sperm DNA Integrity

The sperm DNA fragmentation index (SDF), a marker of DNA damage in sperm, has been advocated as a promising parameter for fertility investigation because the biologic variation in sperm DNA damage is less than traditional semen parameters [73, 219, 220, 273]. Increased sperm DNA fragmentation has been associated with poor pregnancy rates in both natural conception and assisted reproductive techniques, and emerging evidence indicates that men with varicocele have higher levels of sperm DNA damage than their fertile counterparts [273, 274]. It has been also reported that microsurgical varicocelectomy decrease sperm DNA damage and increase chromatin compaction [24, 32, 33, 35]. In a meta-analysis exploring the relationship between varicocele and sperm DNA fragmentation, seven studies determined the magnitude of sperm DNA damage caused by varicocele while six studies evaluated the efficacy of varicocelectomy to alleviate such damage. The overall estimate showed that patients with varicocele have significantly higher sperm DNA damage than controls, with a mean difference of 9.84 % (95 % CI 9.19 to 10.49;

$p<0.00001$). Varicocelectomy improved sperm DNA integrity, with a mean difference of -3.37% (95% CI -4.09 to -2.65; $p<0.00001$) [177].

Improvement in sperm DNA integrity after varicocele repair adds to the evidence supporting the beneficial role of varicocele treatment on spermatogenesis.

Effect on Pregnancy Rates

Natural Pregnancy

In the absence of sufficient large randomized controlled studies with appropriately selected patients, investigators have turned to meta-analysis of the available literature to discern the role of varicocele ligation in male factor infertility, as shown in Table 8.2. In 2004, a Cochrane review [242] concluded that varicocele repair for otherwise unexplained infertility could not be recommended. This conclusion was based on a meta-analysis of eight RCTs showing an odds ratio of only 1.1 favoring treatment over no treatment (95% CI: 0.73–1.68). Although these results received considerable attention and had shaped practice patterns, there were serious methodological inconsistencies in this aforementioned study. Among the included RCTs, three of them evaluated men with subclinical varicocele. As will be described in later ...sections??, men with subclinical varicoceles do not meet the current selection criteria for varicocele repair. Another aspect that deserves attention is the fact that two included studies evaluated men with normal semen analysis. Hence, most of the included studies assessed patients who did not meet the criteria for varicocele repair according to the recommendations of various specialty societies, such as the American Urological Association (AUA), American Society of Reproductive Medicine (ASRM) and the European Association of Urology (EAU) [243] (see Chap. 11).

Ficarra et al. [181] repeated this aforesaid Cochrane review, but excluded those aforementioned studies in which men with normal semen parameters or subclinical varicoceles had been treated. As a result, only three trials including a total of 237 patients were analyzed. The authors showed pregnancy rates were higher in treated (36.4%) compared with untreated patients (20%; $p=0.009$). In 2007, Marmar et al. [182] corroborated the results of Ficarra et al. in a meta-analysis that included RCTs and observational studies involving infertile men with palpable varicocele and abnormal semen parameters. In their study, varicocelectomy significantly improved the odds for natural pregnancy (odds ratio: 2.63–2.87; 95% CI: 1.60–4.33) compared with observation or medical therapy.

Recently in 2012, the Cochrane Institute published a revised meta-analysis on the effects of varicocelectomy in subfertility. The meta-analysis included ten RCTs involving 894 men. None of the studies reported a live birth. The combined fixed-effect odds ratio (OR) of the 10 studies for the outcome of pregnancy was 1.47 (95% CI: 1.05–2.05) favoring the intervention. The number needed to treat for an additional pregnancy was 17, suggesting benefit of varicocele treatment over ex-

Table 8.2 Meta-analysis of studies evaluating the effect of varicocele treatment on natural pregnancy rates

Study	Study population	Design	Intervention	Outcome	Comment
Cochrane 2004 [242]	607	Eight RCT reporting pregnancy rates as an outcome measure	Surgical ligation or radiological embolization of the internal spermatic vein and untreated groups	Peto odds ratio (OR) of the eight studies was 1.10 (95%CI 0.73–1.68), indicating no benefit of varicoceles treatment over expectant management in subfertile couples in whom varicoceles is the only abnormal finding in the man	Two trials involving clinical varicoceles included some men with normal semen analysis. Three studies specifically addressed only men with subclinical varicoceles
Ficarra et al. 2006 [181]	Group 1: 120 infertile with varicocele who underwent surgical repair; Group 2: 117 men with untreated varicocele	Three RCT reporting pregnancy rates as an outcome measure	Surgical ligation or radiological embolization of the internal spermatic vein and untreated groups	Significant increase in pregnancy rate (PR) in patients who underwent varicocele treatment (36.4%) compared with the control group (20%) ($p=0.009$)	Revaluation of Cochrane meta-analysis (2004) excluding men with normal semen and subclinical varicocele
Marmar et al. 2007 [182]	396 infertile men underwent varicocele repair (group 1); 174 untreated men with varicocele and infertility (Group 2)	Two RCTs and three observational studies	Surgical varicocelectomy compared with no or medical treatment for palpable varicocele and at least one abnormal semen parameter	Significant increase in pregnancy rate (PR) in patients who underwent varicocele treatment (33.3%) compared with the control group (15%); Odds of natural pregnancy after surgical varicocelectomy, compared with no or medical treatment were 2.87 (95% confidence interval [CI], 1.33–6.20) with use of a random-effects model or 2.63 (95% CI, 1.60–4.33) with use of a fixed-effects model	The number needed to treat was 5.7 (95% CI, 4.4–9.5)

Table 8.2 (continued)

Study	Study population	Design	Intervention	Outcome	Comment
Baazzeem [284]	380	Four RCTs reporting on pregnancy outcome after repair of clinical varicoceles in oligozoospermic men	Surgical ligation and untreated groups	Using the random effect model, the combined odds ratio was 2.23 (95 % confidence interval [CI], 0.86–5.78; $p = 0.091$), indicating that varicocelectomy is moderately superior to observation, but the effect is not statistically significant	Authors identified 22, 17, and 5 prospective studies reporting on sperm concentration, total motility, and progressive motility, respectively, before and after repair of clinical varicocele. The random effect model combined improvement in sperm concentration was 12.32 million sperm per milliliter (95 % CI, 9.45–15.19; $p < 0.0001$). The random effect model combined improvement in sperm total and progressive motility were 10.86 % (95 % CI, 7.07–14.65; $p < 0.0001$) and 9.69 % (95 % CI, 4.86–14.52; $p = 0.003$), respectively
Cochrane (2012) [275]	894	Ten RCTs reporting pregnancy rates as an outcome measure	Surgical ligation or radiological embolization of the internal spermatic vein and untreated groups	The combined fixed-effect OR was 1.47 (95 % CI: 1.05–2.05, very low quality evidence), favoring the intervention. The number needed to treat for an additional beneficial outcome was 17, suggesting benefit of varicocele treatment over expectant management for pregnancy rate in subfertile couples in whom varicocele in the man was the only abnormal finding	Subgroup analysis after exclusion of the studies including men with normal semen analysis and subclinical varicocele (five studies) revealed favorable effect of treatment (combined OR: 2.39; 95 % CI: 1.56–3.66; high statistical heterogeneity I(2) = 67%). The number needed to treat for an additional beneficial outcome was 7

RCT randomized controlled trial, *OR* odds ratio, *CI* confidence interval pectant management in subfertile couples in whom varicocele was the only abnormal finding. Omission of studies that included men with normal semen analysis and subclinical varicocele, some of which had had semen analysis improvement as the primary outcome rather than live birth or pregnancy rate, was the subject of a planned subgroup analysis. The outcome of the subgroup analysis (five studies) also favored treatment, with a combined OR of 2.39 (95 % CI 1.56–3.66). The number needed to treat for an additional beneficial outcome was 7. The evidence was suggestive rather than conclusive, as the main analysis was subject to fairly high statistical heterogeneity ($I^2 = 67\%$), and findings were no longer significant when a random-effects model was used or when analysis was restricted to higher quality studies. The authors concluded that there is evidence suggesting that treatment of a varicocele in men from couples with otherwise unexplained subfertility may improve a couple's chance of pregnancy. However, the authors commented about the quality of the available evidence being very low, and that more research is needed with live birth or pregnancy rate as the primary outcome [275].

Assisted Conception

Assisted reproductive technology (ART), including *in vitro* fertilization (IVF) and intracytoplasmic sperm injection (ICSI), is routinely used to treat male factor infertility. Because of the success of ART, the optimal method to achieve pregnancy in cases involving treatable causes of male infertility has been debated. Decision analysis-based comparisons of ART and varicocelectomy suggest that varicocele repair is more cost-effective than the use of ART in men with impaired semen parameters [255, 262], as discussed in Chap. 10. Moreover, the indication of varicocele repair prior to IVF/ICSI may be considered in certain circumstances. Men with non-obstructive azoospermia (NOA) and favorable testicular histopathology may resume minimal sperm production following repair of clinical varicocele [231], as discussed in Chap. 9. Sperm restoration, even if minimal, yields the possibility of IVF/ICSI without the need for sperm retrieval (SR) techniques. It has been shown that for patients who are still azoospermic after varicocelectomy, SR success rates using testicular microdissection sperm extraction, and as a result, the couple's chances of a successful pregnancy may be increased [276].

Varicocelectomy has also a potential to obviate the need for ART or to downstage the level of ART needed to bypass male factor infertility [277]. Recently, it has been shown that treatment of clinical varicocele may also improve the outcomes of assisted reproduction in couples with varicocele-related infertility. Esteves et al. [238] studied 242 infertile men with treated and untreated clinical varicocele who underwent ICSI and found significantly higher live birth rates after ICSI in the group of men who underwent artery and lymphatic-sparing subinguinal microsurgical varicocele repair before ART (46.2 %) as compared to the ones undergoing ICSI in the presence of a clinical varicocele (31.4 %). In their study, the chances of achieving a live birth (OR = 1.87; 95 % CI: 1.08–3.25; $p = 0.03$) by ICSI were significantly increased, while the chances of miscarriage occurrence after obtaining a pregnancy by ICSI were reduced (OR=0.433; 95% CI: 0.22–0.84; p=0.01) had the varicocele been treated before assisted conception.

Does Patient Selection Criteria Affect Outcome?

Studies evaluating predictors for successful varicocele repair indicate that infertile men with either mild/moderate preoperative sperm quality reduction or large varicocele are more likely to achieve postoperative semen parameters improvement [56, 278]. It was also shown that men who achieved a postoperative total motile sperm count greater than 20 million and decreased sperm DNA fragmentation after surgical varicocelectomy were more likely to initiate a pregnancy either naturally or via assisted conception [73, 268]. Conversely, reduced preoperative testicular volume, elevated serum FSH levels, diminished testosterone concentrations, subclinical varicocele, as well as the presence of Y chromosome microdeletions seem to be negative predictors for fertility improvement after surgery [227, 279].

As already discussed, societies' guidelines highlight that varicocele treatment should be offered to men with palpable varicose veins on the physical examination of the scrotum only. Moreover, semen parameters have to be abnormal, and a normal female evaluation or potentially reversible female factor infertility is crucial to allow the possibility of natural conception. In addition to these criteria, there are other preoperative characteristics that may help identify those patients who would achieve the most benefit from varicocele ligation. For instance, it has been suggested that reversal of blood flow in the varicocele during a Valsalva maneuver on ultrasound exam was shown to significantly better predict an improvement in semen parameters than if reversal of flow could not be documented. The same study also noted that men with the largest vein measuring 3 mm or greater on ultrasound showed significant improvement in semen parameters, whereas those with the largest vein less than 3 mm did not. Unfortunately, pregnancy data were not available [280]. In another study, patients with treated bilateral varicoceles had greater improvement in semen parameters than those with unilateral varicocele, albeit an improvement in sperm quality was noted in both groups. Pregnancy rates were also higher in the group with bilateral varicocele repair (49 vs. 36%; $p<0.05$) [281]). Lastly, the individual response after varicocele repair may be also related to the different profile of antioxidant enzymes genotype in infertile men with varicocele. It has been suggested that genetic polymorphisms in the glutathione S-transferase T1 gene may affect individual response to varicocelectomy [282].

In conclusion, conflicting results obtained from different studies attempting to answer to the question of whether or not varicocelectomy improves fertility seems to be due to heterogeneous study designs and, more importantly, patient selection criteria. No definitive randomized prospective clinical trial of sufficient size exists at this time due to the inherent difficulties of establishing such a trial and enrolling infertility patients. In the absence of such a trial, critical assessment of the best quality data available leads to the conclusion that varicocelectomy can benefit appropriately selected infertile men.

Key Points

- Varicocelectomy is believed to improve one or more semen parameters in 65% of the treated subjects. The mean postoperative time for semen improvement and natural pregnancy is approximately 5 and 7 months, respectively.
- A significant attenuation of oxidative stress markers occurs after varicocelectomy, and such effects are firstly seen 1 month after varicocele repair.
- Significant improvement in sperm DNA integrity has been demonstrated in infertile men after varicocele repair.
- Natural pregnancy rates after varicocelectomy when female factors are excluded, are approximately 43% at 1 year and 69% at 2 years follow-up. These figures are dependent on proper selection criteria, such as the presence of a palpable varicocele on the physical examination of the scrotum and abnormal semen parameters.
- Treatment of clinical varicocele may improve the outcomes of assisted reproduction in couples with varicocele-related infertility.

Chapter 9
Varicocele and Azoospermia

Azoospermia is defined as the complete absence of sperm from the ejaculate without implying an underlying cause. This condition is present in approximately 1 % of all men and up to 15 % of infertile men [285, 286]. Azoospermia may result from mechanical blockage occurring anywhere along the reproductive tract, including the vas deferens, epididymis, and ejaculatory duct, but most often it is associated with a spectrum of various severe and untreatable conditions causing an intrinsic testicular impairment, which is termed non-obstructive azoospermia (NOA) [287]. Varicocele is found in 5 % of men with NOA, but its absolute impact on the azoospermic status is still unknown [230]. The advent of assisted reproductive technologies (ART), particularly intracytoplasmic sperm injection (ICSI), has reintroduced the awareness about varicocele with NOA, as improvement in testicular function to obtain viable sperm for ART may be critical for infertile men with NOA.

Genetic evaluation including karyotype and Y chromosome mapping are crucial in the work-up of men with varicocele and azoospermia. Microdeletions of the Y chromosome (YCMD) can be identified in up to 18 % of these men [286]. Molecular diagnosis and subtyping of Y-chromosome microdeletions (YCMD) have been useful markers not only to detect the males in whom NOA is caused by YCMD, but also to counsel the affected patients about their chances of sperm retrieval success. Furthermore, the affected patients should be aware of abnormalities so that they can obtain genetic counseling in order to quantify their risk of transmitting them to their offspring. Finding a microdeletion within the AZFa or AZFb regions practically implies that the chances of SR success are virtually non-existent. Therefore, it would be unreliable to recommend varicocele repair in such cases [288, 289].

A meta-analysis was conducted to assess the impact of surgical repair in 233 men with clinical varicocele and NOA [231]. At an average follow-up of 13 months, motile spermatozoa were detected in 39 % of subjects and pregnancy was successfully attained in approximately 26 % of men with sperm in the ejaculate, 60 % unassisted (14 cases), and 40 % with in vitro fertilization techniques. Postoperative mean sperm density and percent sperm motility were 1.6 million and 20 %, respectively. Testicular histopathology was the single predictor of success. Success rates in patients with maturation arrest (42.1 %) or hypospermatogenesis (HS) (54.5 %) were

© The Author(s) 2016

A. Hamada et al., *Varicocele and Male Infertility,* SpringerBriefs in Reproductive Biology, DOI 10.1007/978-3-319-24936-0_9

significantly higher than in those with Sertoli-cell-only (SCO) (11.3%, $p < 0.001$ in both groups). These results indicated that biopsy-proven hypospermatogenesis and maturation arrest (MA) were significantly more likely to correlate with finding sperm in the ejaculate than Sertoli-cell only (odds ratio 9.4; CI 95% 3.2–27.3) [231]. Since a gradual decline in spermatogenesis and return to azoospermia have been reported in up to 55.5% of patients 1 year after surgery, semen cryopreservation may be recommended following initial improvement after surgery because the beneficial effects of varicocele repair in the recovery of spermatogenesis may be only temporary [290)].

The aforementioned data was corroborated by another meta-analysis compiling five studies and 90 patients with varicocele and NOA. Testis biopsy revealed hypospermatogenesis in 30 out of 90 men (33%), maturation arrest in 26 out of 90 (29%) and Sertoli-cell-only in 34 out of 90 (38%) [291]. The successful appearance of spermatozoa in the ejaculate after varicocele repair was significantly higher in men classified as having hypospermatogenesis or maturation arrest than those with Sertoli-cell-only (18 out of 30 vs one out of 34, $p = 0.001$; 12 out of 26 vs one out of 34, $p = 0.002$), respectively. The success rate of varicocele repair did not differ when hypospermatogenesis was compared with maturation arrest (18 out of 30 vs 12 out of 26, $p = 0.65$) [291]. Furthermore, the group of men with hypospermatogenesis or maturation arrest at spermatid stage achieved higher success (13 out of 26) after surgery compared with the group of men with maturation arrest at early spermatocyte or Sertoli cell only (0 out of 18). The difference was statistically significant ($p = 0.001$) [291].

The informative nature of the histopathology results in deciding to pursue a varicocele repair would allow for evidence? that about 50% of the men with NOA avoided an unnecessary varicocelectomy. However, the risks of performing a diagnostic testicular biopsy with the sole purpose of histopathology evaluation may outweigh the benefits, as biopsies could remove focal areas of spermatogenesis that will jeopardize future retrieval attempts. Whenever a biopsy is carried out, caution should be taken to excise minimal tissue. Examination of wet specimens for the presence of sperm would allow cryopreservation to be offered. In addition, a meticulous histopathology evaluation would allow to differentiate pure SCO pattern from the cases in which focal spermatogenesis existed.

Although motile ejaculated sperm is preferred for ICSI, persistent azoospermia after varicocele repair is still a potential problem and surgical sperm retrieval (SR) before ICSI will be inevitable for many individuals [290]. Nevertheless, since higher fertilization rates and better ICSI outcomes when fresh, motile, ejaculated sperm are used compared with sperm provided by testicular biopsy or microsurgical testicular sperm extraction, contemplating varicocele repair to help with the appearance of viable sperm in the ejaculates of men with NOA remains an attractive option [292].

As far as sperm retrieval is concerned, comparative studies involving varicocele-treated and untreated individuals are scarce. In one study, SR rates were similar (60%) in azoospermic men who underwent varicocele repair versus those who did not [293]. Nevertheless, others suggested a beneficial role of intervention. Inci et al. [276] studying a group of 96 men observed that SR success was 2.6 fold higher in treated compared with untreated men (53 *vs.* 30%, OR: 2.63, 95% CI: 1.05–6.60; $p = 0.03$). In another study involving 66 men, Haydardedeoglu et al. [294] reported higher SR success in men who had varicocele repair prior to SR (61%) compared with untreated men (38%; $p < 0.01$).

Although an argument can be made that a control group would remain azoospermic, it is not rare to observe that NOA men occasionally ejaculate small quantities of motile sperm even without any intervention.

In conclusion, the limited available evidence precludes a firm conclusion about the role of varicocele and the benefits of its repair in men with NOA. Until a consensus is reached on the optimal management approach to infertile men with NOA and varicocele, it seems reliable to offer varicocele repair to men with hypospermatogenesis and maturation arrest provided YCMD involving the subregions AZFa and AZFb have been excluded. Men with SCO pattern and those who failed to have sperm in their ejaculates after varicocele repair can be counseled to pursue surgical sperm retrieval. Along these lines, it has been our routine to offer microsurgical repair of varicoceles before sperm retrieval, particularly to young men (<35 years) with large bilateral varicoceles (Grades 2 and 3) after proper counseling [273].

Key Points

- Varicocele is found in 5% of men with non-obstructive azoospermia.
- As crucial part of in the work-up of azoospermic men with varicocele, genetic evaluation is pre-requisite including karyotype and Y chromosome mapping. Genetic testing and counseling is important to select the patients who might benefit from varicocele repair, and raise parental awareness about possibility of transmission of any genetic alteration to biological offspring.
- Microdeletions of the Y chromosome (YCMD) can be identified in up to 18% of these men. YCMD within the AZFa or AZFb subregions virtually implies that there are no chances of sperm retrieval success. Therefore, it would be practically unwise to recommend varicocele repair in such cases.
- Testicular histopathology was the single main determinant for successful appearance of the spermatozoa in the ejaculate and for successful pregnancy outcomes.
- A firm recommendation about the role of varicocele repair in men with NOA is still to be determined. There is critical need for randomized controlled trials to examine the potential advantages of varicocele repair in men with NOA.

Chapter 10
Cost-Effectiveness of Varicocele Treatment

Cost-effectiveness analysis (CEA) is a form of economic analysis that compares the relative costs and outcomes (effects) of two or more courses of action. The cost-effectiveness of a therapeutic intervention is the ratio of the cost of the intervention to a relevant measure of its effect. Cost refers to the resources expended for the intervention, usually measured in monetary, terms while the measure of effects depends on the intervention being considered.

In the context of infertility related to varicocele, the relevant outcome is pregnancy or live birth per group of treated couples. Considering that most infertility treatments are partially or not covered by insurance plans the cost of treatment will be influenced by the payer source. An analysis of various treatment strategies including observation, varicocele repair, intrauterine insemination (IUI), and *in vitro* fertilization (IVF), either as a first option or after failures of other options showed that the cost-effectiveness depended on the payer source [295]. In addition, various other costs can be considered beyond the direct cost of medical care, including costs of multiple gestation and complications, which may impact the usefulness of such models.

In 1997, Schlegel reported cost estimates per delivery to evaluate the cost-effectiveness of ART by use of IVF with intracytoplasmic sperm injection (ICSI) as a primary treatment for varicocele-associated infertility in the United States [296]. The cost per delivery with ICSI was found to be 89,091 US dollars (USD) (95 % CI, 78,720–99,462), whereas the cost per delivery after varicocelectomy was 26,268 USD (95 % CI, 19,138–44,656). The authors' data indicated that treatment of varicocele-associated infertility by varicocelectomy is more cost-effective than primary treatment with ART.

Penson et al. [295] also performed a cost-effectiveness analysis of treatment for varicocele-related infertility studying 4 treatment strategies, namely observation, surgical varicocelectomy followed by in vitro fertilization (IVF) if unsuccessful, gonadotropin-stimulated intrauterine insemination (IUI) followed by IVF if unsuccessful, and immediate IVF . The main outcome measure was incremental cost per live delivery of any number of newborns. Immediate IVF cost more per live delivery and was less effective than varicocelectomy followed by IVF if unsuccessful,

© The Author(s) 2016
A. Hamada et al., *Varicocele and Male Infertility,* SpringerBriefs in Reproductive
Biology, DOI 10.1007/978-3-319-24936-0_10

or IUI followed by IVF if unsuccessful. When electing the latter 2 procedures, the preferred approach depended on the payer. IUI followed by IVF was the most cost-effective approach from the patient's perspective, as its final cost was a few hundred dollars less than varicocele repair followed by IVF [295]. From the healthcare payer perspective, however, each additional live birth that resulted from electing IUI/IVF over varicocelectomy/IVF cost $561,423.

Later in 2005, Meng et al. [297] reported decision analysis models for infertile men seeking paternity with varicocele in which cost of interventions were based on institutional data in the United States. The first decision was the choice between varicocelectomy and ART, and the cost per pregnancy was the end point for comparing the outcomes. In the authors' institution, of all patients, 36.6% of couples achieved natural pregnancy after surgery, but the probability varied according to preoperative total motile count. The pregnancy rate for a single ICSI cycle and 4 IUI cycles was assumed to be 30 and 32%, respectively. Overall, surgical repair was more cost-effective than ART. However, the authors noted that surgical treatment was more cost-effective than ART in certain cases of varicocele- associated infertility. If in a surgeon's experience men with a less severely-impaired preoperative motile sperm count (greater than 10 million motile sperm) cannot achieve a 45% pregnancy rate after surgery, ART can be more cost-effective. This is largely due to the relatively inexpensive IUI procedure for which such couples may qualify. On the contrary, if a surgeon can achieve a greater than 14% pregnancy rate in men with more severe impairment in semen quality (less than 10 million motile sperm), varicocele repair is more cost-effective since these couples generally require ICSI instead of IUI to overcome infertility. The authors however, neither provided data about duration of follow up and time to achieve pregnancy, nor considered other factors such as the number of children desired, the social and monetary costs of intervention in the female partner, the cost of time lost from work or the costs attributable to procedural complications and multiple gestations.

In Korea, Kim [298] suggested that the cost per delivery with ICSI was approximately 16,382,448 Korea Won (KRW) (14,893 USD), and the cost per delivery after varicocelectomy was 11,587,675 KRW (10,534 USD). However, under their national health insurance system, the patient's co-payment after varicocelectomy was 5,258,106 KRW (4780 USD) and 14,977,969 KRW (13,616 USD) after ICSI. These authors advocated varicocelectomy as the first-line infertility treatment because it was more cost-effective compared to ART.

Although most cost-effectiveness studies favor varicocelectomy over assisted reproduction, there are factors that cannot be assigned a monetary value but may be very significant to a given couple. Some couples value the immediacy of ART over the time required for natural conception while others feel that there is a premium on conceiving by the 'most natural' means possible that influence their decision for varicocele repair.

Key Points

1. The cost-effectiveness of these various treatment options for varicocele is a vital issue considering that infertility treatments are often not covered by insurance plans and therefore may be an 'out-of-pocket' expense to the patient.
2. Most studies favor varicocelectomy over assisted reproduction even without accounting for the beneficial effect of varicocelectomy beyond the treatment period.
3. Immediate IVF cost more per live delivery and was less effective than varicocelectomy/IVF or IUI/IVF.
4. An analysis of various treatment strategies including observation, varicocele repair, IUI, and immediate IVF, with IVF offered after failures of other options, showed that the most cost-effective approach depended on the payer source whether the healthcare payer or patient's perspective.

Chapter 11
Guidelines and Best Practice Statements for the Evaluation and Management of Infertile Adult and Adolescent Males with Varicocele

With the continuous growth of medical knowledge and the need to improve efficiency in the diagnosis and treatment of medical-related conditions, the role for and utility of clinical guidelines have received increasing attention. Medical specialty associations have created guidelines and best practice statements to better assist practicing physicians in the management of infertile males with varicocele.

The aim of guidelines and best practice statements for the management of the infertile male and adolescents with varicocele is to help urologists and other health care clinicians to promote quality healthcare and discourage potentially harmful or ineffective interventions. Among urologists and other professionals in reproductive medicine, the three most commonly utilized guidelines for the evaluation and management of infertile males with varicocele are as follows: (i) The American Urological Association (AUA) Best Practice Statement for the Evaluation of the Infertile Male (American Urological Association Education and Research 2010) [299], (ii) Report on Varicocele and Infertility: a Committee Opinion. (Practice Committee of American Society for Reproductive Medicine 2014) [300], and (iii) The European Association of Urology (EAU) Guidelines on Male Infertility [301]. In addition, the EAU Guidelines on Pediatric Urology includes a dedicated chapter on the diagnosis and management of children and adolescent varicocele [302].

Several consensus opinions exist from other countries, but the aforementioned guidelines have been regularly and systematically updated and are therefore considered evolving projects based on the best clinical evidence available. These guidelines are endorsed and adopted by some of the most important specialty societies in urology/reproductive medicine worldwide, and they fulfill the criteria of "Clinical Practice Guidelines" developed by the Institute of Medicine (Institute of Medicine 2011 [303]). According to the Institute of Medicine, clinical practice guidelines should be developed based on a systematic review of evidence, and the final document must include statements and recommendations intended to optimize patient care and assist physicians and/or other health care practitioners and patients to make decisions about appropriate health care for specific clinical circumstances.

Although these guidelines attempt to translate best evidence into practice, there are significant differences in the methods of guidelines' development, data

© The Author(s) 2016
A. Hamada et al., *Varicocele and Male Infertility,* SpringerBriefs in Reproductive Biology, DOI 10.1007/978-3-319-24936-0_11

Table 11.1 Levels of evidence and grades of recommendation as used in the European Association of Urology Clinical Guidelines

Levels of evidence	
1a	Evidence obtained from meta-analysis of randomized trials
1b	Evidence obtained from at least one randomized trial
2a	Evidence obtained from one well-designed controlled study without randomization
2b	Evidence obtained from at least one other type of well-designed quasi-experimental study
3	Evidence obtained from well-designed non-experimental studies, such as comparative studies, correlation studies and case reports
4	Evidence obtained from expert committee reports or opinions or clinical experience of respected authorities
Rating scheme for the grade of recommendations	
A	Based on clinical studies of good quality and consistency addressing the specific recommendations and including at least one randomized trial
B	Based on well-conducted clinical studies, but without randomized clinical trials
C	Made despite the absence of directly applicable clinical studies of good quality

collection and analysis, which influence both the quality and strength of statements made and recommendations provided. Of them, only the EAU guidelines provide evidence-based levels for the recommendations given, as shown in Table 11.1 [301]. However, most recommendations were derived from non-randomized clinical trials, retrospective studies and expert opinion, thus suggesting ample opportunities for research and future incorporation of higher quality standards in male infertility care.

Guidelines statements are not intended to be used as a 'legal standard' against which physicians should be measured but rather serve to provide a framework of standardized care while maintaining clinical autonomy and physician judgment. Although guidelines are intended to offer advantages in standardization of care, improvement in efficiency, enhanced research opportunities, and creation of a cost-effective diagnosis/treatment algorithm, many physicians opt not to adopt guidelines for various reasons, including financial, technical and personal factors. Despite these limitations, a combination of a guideline-based management combined with physician judgment is likely to represent the most prevailing standard of care [304].

Diagnosis

AUA and ASRM Guidelines

According to the AUA and ASRM, a palpable varicocele can be detected in infertile men in erect position and feels like a "bag of worms" and it disappears or very significantly diminishes in size when the patient is recumbent. If the varicocele is not clearly palpable, a repeat examination is advised in erect position with Valsalva maneuver.

Only clinically-palpable varicoceles have been evidently associated with infertility. Varicoceles are characteristically graded on a scale of 1–3, in which grade 3 is visually inspected, grade 2 is easily palpable, and grade 1 is only palpable with Valsalva maneuver [185]. These definitions are rather equivocal and subjective definitions, as what may be easily palpable to one examiner may not be for another. However, there is agreement that varicoceles palpable by most examiners are considered "clinically significant."

Ancillary diagnostic measures, such as scrotal ultrasonography, thermography, Doppler examination, radionuclide scanning, and spermatic venography, should not be used for routine screening and detection of subclinical varicoceles in patients without a palpable abnormality.

Scrotal ultrasonography is indicated for evaluation of a questionable physical examination of the scrotum. Although decisive evidence-based criteria for diagnosis of varicocele are lacking, the current consensus agrees that multiple spermatic veins >2.5–3.0 mm in diameter (at rest and with Valsalva) tend to correlate with the presence of clinically-significant varicoceles [186].

In persistent and recurrent varicocele after surgical repair, spermatic venography is useful to demonstrate the anatomic position of refluxing spermatic veins. Although early studies did not demonstrate a difference in outcome based on varicocele size, more recent data suggest that larger varicoceles may have a greater impact on semen parameters, and correction may result in greater improvement [224].

EAU Guidelines

The EAU guidelines recommends that diagnosis of varicocele is initially made by clinical examination and should be confirmed by color Doppler analysis in the supine and upright position [185, 302].

In children and adolescents, the size of the testis should be evaluated during palpation to detect a smaller testis. To discriminate testicular hypoplasia, the testicular volume is measured by ultrasound examination or by orchidometer. In adolescents, a testis that is smaller by more than 2 mL or 20% compared to the other testis is considered to be hypoplastic [121] (Level of evidence 2). In order to assess testicular injury in adolescents with varicocele, supranormal follicle-stimulating hormone (FSH) and luteinizing hormone (LH) responses to the luteinizing hormone-releasing hormone (LHRH) stimulation test are considered reliable, because histopathological testicular changes have been found in these patients [254, 305].

In centers where treatment is carried out by antegrade or retrograde sclerotherapy or embolization, diagnosis is additionally confirmed by venographic studies.

Clinically, varicocele is graded in the same manner as stated by the AUA/ASRM guidelines. Subclinical varicocele are defined as those not palpable or visible at rest or during Valsalva maneuver, but shown by special tests such as Doppler ultrasound studies.

Treatment

ASRM and AUA Guidelines

Adult Varicocele

Treatment of adult infertile male with varicocele attempting to induce pregnancy is recommended when most or all of the following conditions are met:

i. The varicocele is palpable on physical examination of the scrotum;
ii. The couple has known infertility;
iii. The female partner has normal fertility or a potentially treatable cause of infertility, and time to conception is not a concern;
iv. The male partner has abnormal semen parameters.

Varicocele treatment is not indicated in patients with either normal semen quality, isolated teratozoospermia, or a subclinical varicocele [186]. Furthermore, a man who is not currently attempting to induce conception but has a palpable varicocele, abnormal semen parameters and a desire for future fertility, and/or pain related to the varicocele is also a candidate for varicocele repair.

Young adult males with clinical varicoceles who have normal semen parameters may be at risk for progressive testicular dysfunction and should be offered monitoring with semen analyses every 1–2 years to detect the earliest sign of reduced spermatogenesis. More recently, there is increased evidence that larger varicoceles may impact testosterone production, and some advocate repair in the setting of diminished testosterone levels [296].

Adolescent Varicocele

Adolescent males who have unilateral or bilateral varicocele and objective evidence of testicular hypotrophy ipsilateral to the varicocele may also be considered candidates for varicocele ligation [254, 306–308]. If no reduction in testicular size is evident annual objective measurement of testis size and/or semen analyses to monitor for earliest sign of varicocele-related testicular injury. Varicocele repair may be offered on detection of testicular or semen abnormalities, as catch-up growth has been demonstrated as well as reversal of semen abnormalities; however, data are lacking regarding the impact on future fertility

EAU Guidelines

Adult Varicocele

EAU grade A recommendation indicates that: (i) Varicocele repair should be considered in case of a clinical varicocele, oligozoospermia, infertility duration of >2 years and otherwise unexplained infertility in the couple; (ii) No evidence indicates benefit from varicocele treatment in infertile men who have normal semen analysis or in men with subclinical varicocele. In this situation, varicocele treatment cannot be recommended [257, 284, 309].

Adolescent Varicocele

The EAU guidelines on male infertility recommend varicocele treatment to adolescents with progressive failure of testicular development documented by serial clinical examination (Grade B recommendation). In contrast, the EAU guidelines on pediatric urology indicates that the criteria for varicocelectomy in children and adolescents are as follows:

i. Varicocele associated with a small testis;
ii. Additional testicular condition affecting fertility;
iii. Bilateral palpable varicocele;
iv. Pathological sperm quality (in older adolescents);
v. Symptomatic varicocele.

The latter also states that testicular (left + right) volume loss in comparison with normal testes is a promising indication criterion, once the normal values are available [310]. Repair of a large varicocele, physically or psychologically causing discomfort, may be also considered. Other varicoceles should be followed-up until a reliable sperm analysis can be performed (Level of evidence 4). These aforesaid guidelines adds that there is no evidence that treatment of varicocele at pediatric age will offer a better andrological outcome than an operation performed later (Level of evidence 4).

Treatment Method

ASRM and AUA Guidelines

There are two approaches to varicocele repair: surgery and percutaneous embolization. Surgical repair of a varicocele may be accomplished by various open surgical methods, including retroperitoneal, inguinal, and subinguinal approaches, or by laparoscopy. Percutaneous embolization treatment of a varicocele is accomplished by percutaneous embolization of the refluxing internal spermatic vein(s). None of these methods has been proven superior to the others in its ability to improve fertility, although there are differences in recurrence rates.

EAU Guidelines

Adult Varicocele

Several treatments are available for varicocele. The type of intervention chosen depends mainly on the experience of the therapist. Although laparoscopic varicocelectomy is feasible, it must be justified in terms of cost-effectiveness. Current evidence indicates that microsurgical varicocelectomy is the most effective and least morbid method among the varicocelectomy techniques [257].

Children and Adolescent Varicocele

For surgical ligation, some form of optical magnification (microscopic or laparoscopic magnification) should be used. Lymphatic-sparing varicocelectomy is preferred to prevent hydrocele formation and testicular hypertrophy (Level of evidence 2; Grade B recommendation).

Key Points

The AUA and ASRM guidelines recommendations are as follow:

1. Physical examination in erect position with or without Valsalva maneuver is sufficient to make the diagnosis
2. Use of Doppler US is recommended in equivocal cases.
3. Repair of varicocele in adult men who are attempting to induce pregnancy is recommended when most or all of the following conditions are met: (i) The varicocele is palpable; (ii) The couple has known infertility; (iii) The female partner has normal fertility or a potentially treatable cause of infertility, and time to conception is not a concern; and (iv) The male partner has abnormal semen parameters.
4. Repair of adolescent varicocele is recommended when there is objective evidence of testicular hypotrophy ipsilateral to the varicocele.

The EAU guidelines recommendations are as follows:

1. Clinical diagnosis of varicocele should be confirmed with Doppler study.
2. Varicocele repair should be considered in men with clinical varicocele, oligozoospermia, infertility duration of >2 years and otherwise unexplained infertility in the couple (Level of evidence 1a; grade A recommendation).

3. No evidence indicates benefit from varicocele treatment in infertile men who have normal semen analysis or in men with subclinical varicocele. In this situation, varicocele treatment cannot be recommended (grade A recommendation).

4. Varicocele treatment is recommended in adolescents with progressive failure of testicular development documented by serial clinical examination (grade B recommendation; EAU guidelines on male infertility). It is also recommended by the EAU guidelines on pediatric urology in the following clinical scenarios: (i) Varicocele associated with a small testis; (ii) Additional testicular condition affecting fertility; (iii) Bilateral palpable varicocele; (iv) Pathological sperm quality (in older adolescents); (v) Symptomatic varicocele (Level of evidence 2; Grade B recommendation).

5. For surgical ligation, some form of optical magnification (microscopic or laparoscopic magnification) should be used. Lymphatic-sparing varicocelectomy is preferred to prevent hydrocele formation and testicular hypertrophy (Level of evidence 2; Grade B recommendation).

References

1. Jarow JP, Coburn M, Sigman M. Incidence of varicoceles in men with primary and secondary infertility. Urology. 1996;47(1):73–6. (PubMed PMID: 8560666).
2. Sayfan J, Soffer Y, Orda R. Varicocele treatment: prospective randomized trial of 3 methods. J Urol. 1992;148(5):1447–9. (PubMed PMID: 1433548).
3. Gorelick JI, Goldstein M. Loss of fertility in men with varicocele. Fertil Steril. 1993;59(3):613–6. (PubMed PMID: 8458466).
4. Esteves SC, Miyaoka R, Agarwal A. An update on the clinical assessment of the infertile male. [corrected]. Clinics. 2011;66(4):691–700. (PubMed PMID: 21655766. Pubmed Central PMCID: 3093801).
5. Sylora JA, Pryor JL. Varicocele. Curr Ther Endocrinol Metab. 1994;5:309–14. (PubMed PMID: 7704742).
6. Green KF, Turner TT, Howards SS. Varicocele: reversal of the testicular blood flow and temperature effects by varicocele repair. J Urol. 1984;131(6):1208–11. (PubMed PMID: 6726930).
7. Akbay E, Cayan S, Doruk E, Duce MN, Bozlu M. The prevalence of varicocele and varicocele-related testicular atrophy in Turkish children and adolescents. BJU Int. 2000;86(4):490–3. (PubMed PMID: 10971279).
8. Oster J. Varicocele in children and adolescents. An investigation of the incidence among Danish school children. Scand J Urol Nephrol. 1971;5(1):27–32. (PubMed PMID: 5093090).
9. Vasavada S, Ross J, Nasrallah P, Kay R. Prepubertal varicoceles. Urology. 1997;50(5):774–7. (PubMed PMID: 9372891).
10. Berger OG. Varicocele in adolescence. Clin Pediatr (Phila). 1980;19(12):810–1. (PubMed PMID: 7438659).
11. Steeno OP. Varicocele in the adolescent. Adv Exp Med Biol. 1991;286:295–321. (PubMed PMID: 2042517).
12. Risser WL, Lipshultz LI. Frequency of varicocele in black adolescents. J Adolesc Health Care. 1984;5(1):28–9. (PubMed PMID: 6607247).
13. Kumanov P, Robeva RN, Tomova A. Adolescent varicocele: who is at risk? Pediatrics. 2008;121(1):e53–7. (PubMed PMID: 18166544).
14. Rais A, Zarka S, Derazne E, Tzur D, Calderon-Margalit R, Davidovitch N, et al. Varicocoele among 1 300 000 Israeli adolescent males: time trends and association with body mass index. Andrology. 2013;1(5):663–9. (PubMed PMID: 23970450).
15. Meacham RB, Townsend RR, Rademacher D, Drose JA. The incidence of varicoceles in the general population when evaluated by physical examination, gray scale sonography and color Doppler sonography. J Urol. 1994;151(6):1535–8. (PubMed PMID: 8189565).
16. Comhaire F, Monteyne R, Kunnen M. The value of scrotal thermography as compared with selective retrograde venography of the internal spermatic vein for the diagnosis of "subclinical" varicocele. Fertil Steril. 1976;27(6):694–8. (PubMed PMID: 1278464).

© The Author(s) 2016
A. Hamada et al., *Varicocele and Male Infertility,* SpringerBriefs in Reproductive Biology, DOI 10.1007/978-3-319-24936-0

17. Hirsh AV, Cameron KM, Tyler JP, Simpson J, Pryor JP. The Doppler assessment of vari-
    coceles and internal spermatic vein reflux in infertile men. Br J Urol. 1980;52(1):50–6.
    (PubMed PMID: 7426951).
18. McClure RD, Hricak H. Scrotal ultrasound in the infertile man: detection of subclinical uni-
    lateral and bilateral varicoceles. J Urol. 1986;135(4):711–5. (PubMed PMID: 3514958).
19. Gonda RL Jr., Karo JJ, Forte RA, O'Donnell KT. Diagnosis of subclinical varicocele in infer-
    tility. AJR Am J Roentgenol. 1987;148(1):71–5. (PubMed PMID: 3024475).
20. Kulis T, Kolaric D, Karlovic K, Knezevic M, Antonini S, Kastelan Z. Scrotal infrared digital
    thermography in assessment of varicocele–pilot study to assess diagnostic criteria. Androlo-
    gia. 2012;44 Suppl 1:780–5. (PubMed PMID: 22191852).
21. Atasoy C, Fitoz S. Gray-scale and color Doppler sonographic findings in intratesticular vari-
    cocele. J Clin Ultrasound. 2001;29(7):369–73. (PubMed PMID: 11579398).
22. Ivanissevich O. Left varicocele due to reflux; experience with 4,470 operative cases in forty-
    two years. J Int Coll Surg. 1960;34:742–55. (PubMed PMID: 13718224).
23. Dhabuwala CB, Hamid S, Moghissi KS. Clinical versus subclinical varicocele: improvement
    in fertility after varicocelectomy. Fertil Steril. 1992;57(4):854–7. (PubMed PMID: 1555699).
24. Marsman JW, Schats R. The subclinical varicocele debate. Hum Reprod. 1994;9(1):1–8.
    (PubMed PMID: 8195328).
25. Braedel HU, Steffens J, Ziegler M, Polsky MS, Platt ML. A possible ontogenic etiology for
    idiopathic left varicocele. J Urol. 1994;151(1):62–6. (PubMed PMID: 8254834).
26. Naughton CK, Nangia AK, Agarwal A. Pathophysiology of varicoceles in male infertility.
    Hum Reprod Update. 2001;7(5):473–81. (PubMed PMID: 11556494).
27. Ahlberg NE, Bartley O, Chidekel N. Right and left gonadal veins. An anatomical and statisti-
    cal study. Acta Radiol Diagn (Stockh). 1966;4(6):593–601. (PubMed PMID: 5929114).
28. Nielsen ME, Zderic S, Freedland SJ, Jarow JP. Insight on pathogenesis of varicoceles: rela-
    tionship of varicocele and body mass index. Urology. 2006;68(2):392–6. (PubMed PMID:
    16904459).
29. Chen SS, Huang WJ. Differences in biochemical markers and body mass index between
    patients with and without varicocele. J Chin Med Assoc. 2010;73(4):194–8. (PubMed PMID:
    20457440).
30. Raman JD, Walmsley K, Goldstein M. Inheritance of varicoceles. Urology. 2005;65(6):1186–
    9. (PubMed PMID: 15913726).
31. Di Luigi L, Gentile V, Pigozzi F, Parisi A, Giannetti D, Romanelli F. Physical activity as a
    possible aggravating factor for athletes with varicocele: impact on the semen profile. Hum
    Reprod. 2001;16(6):1180–4. (PubMed PMID: 11387289).
32. Lechter A, Lopez G, Martinez C, Camacho J. Anatomy of the gonadal veins: a reappraisal.
    Surgery. 1991;109(6):735–9. (PubMed PMID: 2042092).
33. Valji K. Endocrine, exocrine and reproductive system. In: Valji K, editor. The practice of
    interventional radiology, with online cases and video. [Internet]. 1st ed. [424]. Philadelphia:
    Elsevier Saunders.
34. Miyaoka R, Esteves SC. A critical appraisal on the role of varicocele in male infertility. Adv
    Urol. 2012;2012:597495. (PubMed PMID: 22162682. Pubmed Central PMCID: 3228353).
35. Sigmund G, Gall H, Bahren W. Stop-type and shunt-type varicoceles: venographic findings.
    Radiology. 1987;163(1):105–10. (PubMed PMID: 3547489).
36. Cvitanic OA, Cronan JJ, Sigman M, Landau ST. Varicoceles: postoperative prevalence–a
    prospective study with color Doppler US. Radiology. 1993;187(3):711–4. (PubMed PMID:
    8497618).
37. Shafik A, Moftah A, Olfat S, Mohi-el-Din M, el-Sayed A. Testicular veins: anatomy and role
    in varicocelogenesis and other pathologic conditions. Urology. 1990;35(2):175–82. (PubMed
    PMID: 2106185).
38. Mohseni MJ, Nazari H, Amini E, Javan-Farazmand N, Baghayee A, Farzi H, et al. Shunt-type
    and stop-type varicocele in adolescents: prognostic value of these two different hemody-
    namic patterns. Fertil Steril. 2011;96(5):1091–6. (PubMed PMID: 21924715).

39. Gat Y, Gornish M, Chakraborty J, Perlow A, Levinger U, Pasqualotto F. Azoospermia and maturation arrest: malfunction of valves in erect poster of humans leads to hypoxia in sperm production site. Andrologia. 2010;42(6):389–94. (PubMed PMID: 21105890).

40. Mali WP, Oei HY, Arndt JW, Kremer J, Coolsaet BL, Schuur K. Hemodynamics of the varicocele. Part I. Correlation among the clinical, phlebographic and scintigraphic findings. J Urol. 1986;135(3):483–8. (PubMed PMID: 3944891).

41. Kim SH, Park JH, Han MC, Paick JS. Embolization of the internal spermatic vein in varicocele: significance of venous pressure. Cardiovasc Intervent Radiol. 1992;15(2):102–6; discussion 6–7. (PubMed PMID: 1571922).

42. Carl P, Stark L, Ouzoun N, Reindl P. Venous pressure in idiopathic varicocele. Eur Urol. 1993;24(2):214–20. (PubMed PMID: 8375442).

43. Kim SH, Cho SW, Kim HD, Chung JW, Park JH, Han MC. Nutcracker syndrome: diagnosis with Doppler US. Radiology. 1996;198(1):93–7. (PubMed PMID: 8539413).

44. Nishimura Y, Fushiki M, Yoshida M, Nakamura K, Imai M, Ono T, et al. Left renal vein hypertension in patients with left renal bleeding of unknown origin. Radiology. 1986;160(3):663–7. (PubMed PMID: 3737903).

45. Unlu M, Orguc S, Serter S, Pekindil G, Pabuscu Y. Anatomic and hemodynamic evaluation of renal venous flow in varicocele formation using color Doppler sonography with emphasis on renal vein entrapment syndrome. Scand J Urol Nephrol. 2007;41(1):42–6. (PubMed PMID: 17366101).

46. Takebayashi S, Ueki T, Ikeda N, Fujikawa A. Diagnosis of the nutcracker syndrome with color Doppler sonography: correlation with flow patterns on retrograde left renal venography. AJR Am J Roentgenol. 1999;172(1):39–43. (PubMed PMID: 9888735).

47. Park SJ, Lim JW, Cho BS, Yoon TY, Oh JH. Nutcracker syndrome in children with orthostatic proteinuria: diagnosis on the basis of Doppler sonography. J Ultrasound Med. 2002;21(1):39–45; quiz 6. (PubMed PMID: 11794401).

48. Coolsaet BL. The varicocele syndrome: venography determining the optimal level for surgical management. J Urol. 1980;124(6):833–9. (PubMed PMID: 7441834).

49. Mali WP, Oei HY, Arndt JW, Kremer J, Coolsaet BL, Schuur K. Hemodynamics of the varicocele. Part II. Correlation among the results of renocaval pressure measurements, varicocele scintigraphy and phlebography. J Urol. 1986;135(3):489–93. (PubMed PMID: 3944892).

50. Fretz PC, Sandlow JI. Varicocele: current concepts in pathophysiology, diagnosis, and treatment. Urol Clin North Am. 2002;29(4):921–37. (PubMed PMID: 12516762).

51. Zerhouni EA, Siegelman SS, Walsh PC, White RI. Elevated pressure in the left renal vein in patients with varicocele: preliminary observations. J Urol. 1980;123(4):512–3. (PubMed PMID: 7365887).

52. Okada M, Tsuzuki K, Ito S. Diagnosis of the nutcracker phenomenon using two-dimensional ultrasonography. Clin Nephrol. 1998;49(1):35–40. (PubMed PMID: 9491284).

53. Graif M, Hauser R, Hirshebein A, Botchan A, Kessler A, Yabetz H. Varicocele and the testicular-renal venous route: hemodynamic Doppler sonographic investigation. J Ultrasound Med. 2000;19(9):627–31. (PubMed PMID: 10972559).

54. Gat Y, Gornish M, Navon U, Chakraborty J, Bachar GN, Ben-Shlomo I. Right varicocele and hypoxia, crucial factors in male infertility: fluid mechanics analysis of the impaired testicular drainage system. Reprod Biomed Online. 2006;13(4):510–5. (PubMed PMID: 17007671).

55. Gat Y, Zukerman Z, Chakraborty J, Gornish M. Varicocele, hypoxia and male infertility. Fluid mechanics analysis of the impaired testicular venous drainage system. Hum Reprod. 2005;20(9):2614–9. (PubMed PMID: 15932914).

56. Schlesinger MH, Wilets IF, Nagler HM. Treatment outcome after varicocelectomy. A critical analysis. Urol Clin North Am. 1994;21(3):517–29. (PubMed PMID: 8059505).

57. Hamada A, Esteves SC, Agarwal A. Insight into oxidative stress in varicocele-associated male infertility: part 2. Nat Rev Urol. 2013;10(1):26–37. (PubMed PMID: 23165400).

58. Griveau JF, Le Lannou D. Reactive oxygen species and human spermatozoa: physiology and pathology. Int J Androl. 1997;20(2):61–9. (PubMed PMID: 9292315).

59. Ghabili K, Shoja MM, Agutter PS, Agarwal A. Hypothesis: intracellular acidification con-
    tributes to infertility in varicocele. Fertil Steril. 2009;92(1):399–401. (PubMed PMID:
    18692793).

60. Agarwal A, Prabakaran S, Allamaneni SS. Relationship between oxidative stress, varicocele
    and infertility: a meta-analysis. Reprod Biomed Online. 2006;12(5):630–3. (PubMed PMID:
    16790111).

61. Mitropoulos D, Deliconstantinos G, Zervas A, Villiotou V, Dimopoulos C, Stavrides J. Ni-
    tric oxide synthase and xanthine oxidase activities in the spermatic vein of patients with
    varicocele: a potential role for nitric oxide and peroxynitrite in sperm dysfunction. J Urol.
    1996;156(6):1952–8. (PubMed PMID: 8911364).

62. Allamaneni SS, Naughton CK, Sharma RK, Thomas AJ, Jr., Agarwal A. Increased seminal
    reactive oxygen species levels in patients with varicoceles correlate with varicocele grade but
    not with testis size. Fertil Steril. 2004;82(6):1684–6. (PubMed PMID: 15589881).

63. Koksal IT, Tefekli A, Usta M, Erol H, Abbasoglu S, Kadioglu A. The role of reactive oxygen
    species in testicular dysfunction associated with varicocele. BJU Int. 2000;86(4):549–52.
    (PubMed PMID: 10971290).

64. Mostafa T, Anis TH, El-Nashar A, Imam H, Othman IA. Varicocelectomy reduces reactive
    oxygen species levels and increases antioxidant activity of seminal plasma from infertile men
    with varicocele. Int J Androl. 2001;24(5):261–5. (PubMed PMID: 11554982).

65. Cervellione RM, Cervato G, Zampieri N, Corroppolo M, Camoglio F, Cestaro B, et al.
    Effect of varicocelectomy on the plasma oxidative stress parameters. J Pediatr Surg.
    2006;41(2):403–6. (PubMed PMID: 16481259).

66. Shiraishi K, Naito K. Generation of 4-hydroxy-2-nonenal modified proteins in testes pre-
    dicts improvement in spermatogenesis after varicocelectomy. Fertil Steril. 2006;86(1):233–5.
    (PubMed PMID: 16730723).

67. Saleh RA, Agarwal A, Sharma RK, Said TM, Sikka SC, Thomas AJ Jr. Evaluation of
    nuclear DNA damage in spermatozoa from infertile men with varicocele. Fertil Steril.
    2003;80(6):1431–6. (PubMed PMID: 14667879).

68. Chen SS, Huang WJ, Chang LS, Wei YH. 8-hydroxy-2'-deoxyguanosine in leukocyte DNA
    of spermatic vein as a biomarker of oxidative stress in patients with varicocele. J Urol.
    2004;172(4 Pt 1):1418–21. (PubMed PMID: 15371859).

69. Sadek A, Almohamdy AS, Zaki A, Aref M, Ibrahim SM, Mostafa T. Sperm chromatin
    condensation in infertile men with varicocele before and after surgical repair. Fertil Steril.
    2011;95(5):1705–8. (PubMed PMID: 21292253).

70. Zini A, Blumenfeld A, Libman J, Willis J. Beneficial effect of microsurgical varicocelec-
    tomy on human sperm DNA integrity. Hum Reprod. 2005;20(4):1018–21. (PubMed PMID:
    15608026).

71. Blumer CG, Restelli AE, Giudice PT, Soler TB, Fraietta R, Nichi M, et al. Effect of varico-
    cele on sperm function and semen oxidative stress. BJU Int. 2012;109(2):259–65. (PubMed
    PMID: 21592296).

72. Smith R, Kaune H, Parodi D, Madariaga M, Rios R, Morales I, et al. Increased sperm DNA
    damage in patients with varicocele: relationship with seminal oxidative stress. Hum Reprod.
    2006;21(4):986–93. (PubMed PMID: 16361286).

73. Smit M, Romijn JC, Wildhagen MF, Veldhoven JL, Weber RF, Dohle GR. Decreased sperm
    DNA fragmentation after surgical varicocelectomy is associated with increased pregnancy
    rate. J Urol. 2010;183(1):270–4. (PubMed PMID: 19913801).

74. Dada R, Shamsi MB, Venkatesh S, Gupta NP, Kumar R. Attenuation of oxidative stress &
    DNA damage in varicocelectomy: implications in infertility management. Indian J Med Res.
    2010;132:728–30. (PubMed PMID: 21245622. Pubmed Central PMCID: 3102462).

75. Spano M, Bonde JP, Hjollund HI, Kolstad HA, Cordelli E, Leter G. Sperm chromatin dam-
    age impairs human fertility. The Danish first pregnancy planner study team. Fertil Steril.
    2000;73(1):43–50. (PubMed PMID: 10632410).

76. Zini A, Bielecki R, Phang D, Zenzes MT. Correlations between two markers of sperm DNA integrity, DNA denaturation and DNA fragmentation, in fertile and infertile men. Fertil Steril. 2001;75(4):674–7. (PubMed PMID: 11287017).

77. Goldstein M, Eid JF. Elevation of intratesticular and scrotal skin surface temperature in men with varicocele. J Urol. 1989;142(3):743–5. (PubMed PMID: 2769853).

78. Shiraishi K, Takihara H, Naito K. Testicular volume, scrotal temperature, and oxidative stress in fertile men with left varicocele. Fertil Steril. 2009;91(4 Suppl):1388–91. (PubMed PMID: 18684443).

79. Salisz JA, Kass EJ, Steinert BW. The significance of elevated scrotal temperature in an adolescent with a varicocele. Adv Exp Med Biol. 1991;286:245–51. (PubMed PMID: 2042510. Epub 1991/01/01. eng).

80. Yamaguchi M, Sakatoku J, Takihara H. The application of intrascrotal deep body temperature measurement for the noninvasive diagnosis of varicoceles. Fertil Steril. 1989;52(2):295–301. (PubMed PMID: 2753177. Epub 1989/08/01. eng).

81. Mariotti A, Di Carlo L, Orlando G, Corradini ML, Di Donato L, Pompa P, et al. Scrotal thermoregulatory model and assessment of the impairment of scrotal temperature control in varicocele. Ann Biomed Eng. 2011;39(2):664–73. (PubMed PMID: 20976556. Epub 2010/10/27. eng).

82. Alvarez JG, Storey BT. Spontaneous lipid peroxidation in rabbit and mouse epididymal spermatozoa: dependence of rate on temperature and oxygen concentration. Biol Reprod. 1985;32(2):342–51. (PubMed PMID: 3986267. Epub 1985/03/01. eng).

83. Morgan D, Cherny VV, Murphy R, Xu W, Thomas LL, DeCoursey TE. Temperature dependence of NADPH oxidase in human eosinophils. J Physiol. 2003;550(Pt 2):447–58. (PubMed PMID: 12754316. Epub 2003/05/20. eng).

84. Shin MH, Moon YJ, Seo JE, Lee Y, Kim KH, Chung JH. Reactive oxygen species produced by NADPH oxidase, xanthine oxidase, and mitochondrial electron transport system mediate heat shock-induced MMP-1 and MMP-9 expression. Free Radic Biol Med. 2008;44(4):635–45. (PubMed PMID: 18036352. Epub 2007/11/27. eng).

85. Guo J, Jia Y, Tao SX, Li YC, Zhang XS, Hu ZY, et al. Expression of nitric oxide synthase during germ cell apoptosis in testis of cynomolgus monkey after testosterone and heat treatment. J Androl. 2009;30(2):190–9. (PubMed PMID: 18835830. Epub 2008/10/07. eng).

86. Hadziselimovic F, Herzog B. The importance of both an early orchidopexy and germ cell maturation for fertility. Lancet. 2001;358(9288):1156–7. (PubMed PMID: 11597673. Epub 2001/10/13. eng).

87. Sofikitis N, Miyagawa I. Left adrenalectomy in varicocelized rats does not inhibit the development of varicocele-related physiologic alterations. Int J Fertil Menopausal Stud. 1993;38(4):250–5. (PubMed PMID: 8401685).

88. Nistal M, Gonzalez-Peramato P, Serrano A, Regadera J. [Physiopathology of the infertile testicle. Etiopathogenesis of varicocele]. Arch Esp Urol. 2004;57(9):883–904. (PubMed PMID: 15624389. Fisiopatologia del testiculo infertil. Etiopatogenia del varicocele).

89. Marmar JL. The pathophysiology of varicoceles in the light of current molecular and genetic information. Human Reprod Update. 2001;7(5):461–72. (PubMed PMID: 11556493).

90. Tilki D, Kilic E, Tauber R, Pfeiffer D, Stief CG, Tauber R, et al. The complex structure of the smooth muscle layer of spermatic veins and its potential role in the development of varicocele testis. Eur Urol. 2007;51(5):1402–9; discussion 10. (PubMed PMID: 17113704).

91. Ito H, Fuse H, Minagawa H, Kawamura K, Murakami M, Shimazaki J. Internal spermatic vein prostaglandins in varicocele patients. Fertil Steril. 1982;37(2):218–22. (PubMed PMID: 7060770. Epub 1982/02/01. eng).

92. Adamopoulos DA, Kontogeorgos L, Abrahamian-Michalakis A, Terzis T, Vassilopoulos P. Raised sodium, potassium, and urea concentrations in spermatic venous blood: an additional causative factor in the testicular dysfunction of varicocele? Fertil Steril. 1987;48(2):331–3. (PubMed PMID: 3609346. Epub 1987/08/01. eng).

93. Zhang Z, Yang XY, Cohen DM. Urea-associated oxidative stress and Gadd153/CHOP induction. Am J Physiol. 1999;276(5 Pt 2):F786–93. (PubMed PMID: 10330061).

94. Zhang Z, Dmitrieva NI, Park JH, Levine RL, Burg MB. High urea and NaCl carbonylate proteins in renal cells in culture and in vivo, and high urea causes 8-oxoguanine lesions in their DNA. Proc Natl Acad Sci U S A. 2004;101(25):9491–6. (PubMed PMID: 15190183. Pubmed Central PMCID: 439004).

95. Chen CH, Lee SS, Chen DC, Chien HH, Chen IC, Chu YN, et al. Apoptosis and kinematics of ejaculated spermatozoa in patients with varicocele. J Androl. 2004;25(3):348–53. (PubMed PMID: 15064311).

96. Enciso M, Muriel L, Fernandez JL, Goyanes V, Segrelles E, Marcos M, et al. Infertile men with varicocele show a high relative proportion of sperm cells with intense nuclear damage level, evidenced by the sperm chromatin dispersion test. J Androl. 2006;27(1):106–11. (PubMed PMID: 16400086).

97. Simsek F, Turkeri L, Cevik I, Bircan K, Akdas A. Role of apoptosis in testicular tissue damage caused by varicocele. Arch Esp Urol. 1998;51(9):947–50. (PubMed PMID: 9887572).

98. French DB, Desai NR, Agarwal A. Varicocele repair: does it still have a role in infertility treatment? Curr Opin Obstet Gynecol. 2008;20(3):269–74. (PubMed PMID: 18460942).

99. Ishikawa T, Fujioka H, Ishimura T, Takenaka A, Fujisawa M. Expression of leptin and leptin receptor in the testis of fertile and infertile patients. Andrologia. 2007;39(1):22–7. (PubMed PMID: 17212806).

100. Akkoyunlu G, Erdogru T, Seval Y, Ustunel I, Koksal T, Usta MF, et al. Immunolocalization of glial cell-derived neurotrophic factor (GDNF) and its receptor GFR-alpha1 in varicocele-induced rat testis. Acta Histochem. 2007;109(2):130–7. (PubMed PMID: 17240430).

101. Shiraishi K, Naito K. Increased expression of Leydig cell haem oxygenase-1 preserves spermatogenesis in varicocele. Hum Reprod. 2005;20(9):2608–13. (PubMed PMID: 15878918).

102. Nicotina PA, Romeo C, Arena S, Arena F, Maisano D, Zuccarello B. Immunoexpression of aquaporin-1 in adolescent varicocele testes: possible significance for fluid reabsorption. Urology. 2005;65(1):149–52. (PubMed PMID: 15667881).

103. Ozen IO, Moralioglu S, Vural IM, Ozturk GS, Ozkan MH, Demirtola A, et al. Effects of varicocele on electrical field stimulation-induced biphasic twitch responses in the ipsilateral and contralateral rat vasa deferentia. Eur Surg Res. 2007;39(5):269–74. (PubMed PMID: 17495477).

104. Hendin BN, Kolettis PN, Sharma RK, Thomas AJ Jr., Agarwal A. Varicocele is associated with elevated spermatozoal reactive oxygen species production and diminished seminal plasma antioxidant capacity. J Urol. 1999;161(6):1831–4. (PubMed PMID: 10332447).

105. Pasqualotto FF, Sundaram A, Sharma RK, Borges E Jr., Pasqualotto EB, Agarwal A. Semen quality and oxidative stress scores in fertile and infertile patients with varicocele. Fertil Steril. 2008;89(3):602–7. (PubMed PMID: 17485092).

106. Mostafa T, Anis T, Imam H, El-Nashar AR, Osman IA. Seminal reactive oxygen species-antioxidant relationship in fertile males with and without varicocele. Andrologia. 2009;41(2):125–9. (PubMed PMID: 19260850).

107. Dawes I. Cellular responses to reactive oxygen species. In: Singh KK, editor. Oxidative stress disease and cancer. London: Imperial College Press; 2006. p. 281–308.

108. Baccetti BM, Bruni E, Capitani S, Collodel G, Mancini S, Piomboni P, et al. Studies on varicocele III: ultrastructural sperm evaluation and 18, X and Y aneuploidies. J Androl. 2006;27(1):94–101. (PubMed PMID: 16400084. Epub 2006/01/10. eng).

109. Allen RG, Tresini M. Oxidative stress and gene regulation. Free Radic Biol Med. 2000;28(3):463–99. (PubMed PMID: 10699758. Epub 2000/03/04. eng).

110. Desaint S, Luriau S, Aude JC, Rousselet G, Toledano MB. Mammalian antioxidant defenses are not inducible by H2O2. J Biol Chem. 2004;279(30):31157–63. (PubMed PMID: 15155764. Epub 2004/05/25. eng).

111. Abdel Aziz MT, Mostafa T, Atta H, Kamal O, Kamel M, Hosni H, et al. Heme oxygenase enzyme activity in seminal plasma of oligoasthenoteratozoospermic males with varicocele. Andrologia. 2008;42(4):236–41. (PubMed PMID: 20629646. Epub 2010/07/16. eng).

112. Trum JW, Gubler FM, Laan R, van der Veen F. The value of palpation, varicoscreen contact thermography and colour Doppler ultrasound in the diagnosis of varicocele. Hum Reprod. 1996;11(6):1232–5. (PubMed PMID: 8671430).

113. The influence of varicocele on parameters of fertility in a large group of men presenting to infertility clinics. World Health Organization. Fertil Steril. 1992;57(6):1289–93. (PubMed PMID: 1601152).

114. Chehval MJ, Purcell MH. Deterioration of semen parameters over time in men with untreated varicocele: evidence of progressive testicular damage. Fertil Steril. 1992;57(1):174–7. (PubMed PMID: 1730313).

115. Canales BK, Zapzalka DM, Ercole CJ, Carey P, Haus E, Aeppli D, et al. Prevalence and effect of varicoceles in an elderly population. Urology. 2005;66(3):627–31. (PubMed PMID: 16140091).

116. Kay R, Alexander NJ, Baugham WL. Induced varicoceles in rhesus monkeys. Fertil Steril. 1979;31(2):195–9. (PubMed PMID: 104889).

117. Al-Juburi A, Pranikoff K, Dougherty KA, Urry RL, Cockett AT. Alteration of semen quality in dogs after creation of varicocele. Urology. 1979;13(5):535–9. (PubMed PMID: 442380).

118. Saypol DC, Howards SS, Turner TT, Miller ED, Jr. Influence of surgically induced varicocele on testicular blood flow, temperature, and histology in adult rats and dogs. J Clin Invest. 1981;68(1):39–45. (PubMed PMID: 7251866. Pubmed Central PMCID: 370770).

119. Lyon RP, Marshall S, Scott MP. Varicocele in youth. West J Med. 1983;138(6):832–4. (PubMed PMID: 6613110. Pubmed Central PMCID: 1010829).

120. Steeno O, Knops J, Declerck L, Adimoelja A, van de Voorde H. Prevention of fertility disorders by detection and treatment of varicocele at school and college age. Andrologia. 1976;8(1):47–53. (PubMed PMID: 986121).

121. Diamond DA ZD, Bauer SB, et al. Relationship of varicocele grade and testicular hypotrophy to semen parameters in adolescents. J Urol 2007 178:1584–8.

122. Thomas JC, Elder JS. Testicular growth arrest and adolescent varicocele: does varicocele size make a difference? J Urol. 2002;168(4 Pt 2):1689–91; discussion 91. (PubMed PMID: 12352335).

123. Etriby A, Girgis SM, Hefnawy H, Ibrahim AA. Testicular changes in subfertile males with varicocele. Fertil Steril. 1967;18(5):666–71. (PubMed PMID: 6037454).

124. Dubin L, Hotchkiss RS. Testis biopsy in subfertile men with varicocele. Fertil Steril. 1969;20(1):51–7. (PubMed PMID: 5812532).

125. Ibrahim AA, Awad HA, El-Haggar S, Mitawi BA. Bilateral testicular biopsy in men with varicocele. Fertil Steril. 1977;28(6):663–7. (PubMed PMID: 862978).

126. Cameron DF, Snydle FE, Ross MH, Drylie DM. Ultrastructural alterations in the adluminal testicular compartment in men with varicocele. Fertil Steril. 1980;33(5):526–33. (PubMed PMID: 7371882).

127. Spera G, Medolago-Albani L, Coia L, Morgia C, Gonnelli S, Ghilardi C. Histological, histochemical, and ultrastructural aspects of interstitial tissue from the contralateral testis in infertile men with monolateral varicocele. Arch Androl. 1983;10(1):73–8. (PubMed PMID: 6847308).

128. Cooper TG, Yeung CH. Acquisition of volume regulatory response of sperm upon maturation in the epididymis and the role of the cytoplasmic droplet. Microsc Res Tech. 2003;61(1):28–38. (PubMed PMID: 12672120).

129. Sipila P, Pujianto DA, Shariatmadari R, Nikkila J, Lehtoranta M, Huhtaniemi IT, et al. Differential endocrine regulation of genes enriched in initial segment and distal caput of the mouse epididymis as revealed by genome-wide expression profiling. Biol Reprod. 2006;75(2):240–51. (PubMed PMID: 16641146).

130. Ozturk U, Kefeli M, Asci R, Akpolat I, Buyukalpelli R, Sarikaya S. The effects of experimental left varicocele on the epididymis. Syst Biol Reprod Med. 2008;54(4–5):177–84. (PubMed PMID: 18942025).

131. Zhang QY, Qiu SD, Ma XN, Yu HM, Wu YW. Effect of experimental varicocele on structure and function of epididymis in adolescent rats. Asian J Androl. 2003;5(2):108–12. (PubMed PMID: 12778320).

132. Mahmoud SA, Zahran NM. Electron microscopic study of the left caput epididymal epithelium of adult albino rats in an experimental left varicocele model. Egypt J Histol. 2011;34:483–95.

133. Farias JG, Puebla M, Acevedo A, Tapia PJ, Gutierrez E, Zepeda A, et al. Oxidative stress in rat testis and epididymis under intermittent hypobaric hypoxia: protective role of ascorbate supplementation. J Androl. 2010;31(3):314–21. (PubMed PMID: 20378932).

134. Zaprjanova S, Rashev P, Zasheva D, Martinova Y, Mollova M. Electrophoretic and immunocytochemical analysis of Hsp72 and Hsp73 expression in heat-stressed mouse testis and epididymis. Eur J Obstet Gynecol Reprod Biol. 2013;168(1):54–9. (PubMed PMID: 23352621).

135. Lehtihet M, Arver S, Kalin B, Kvist U, Pousette A. Left-sided grade 3 varicocele may affect the biological function of the epididymis. Scand J Urol. 2014;48(3):284–9. (PubMed PMID: 24354516).

136. Rodriguez-Rigau LJ, Smith KD, Steinberger E. Varicocele and the morphology of spermatozoa. Fertil Steril. 1981;35(1):54–7. (PubMed PMID: 7461154).

137. Zini A, Defreitas G, Freeman M, Hechter S, Jarvi K. Varicocele is associated with abnormal retention of cytoplasmic droplets by human spermatozoa. Fertil Steril. 2000;74(3):461–4. (PubMed PMID: 10973638).

138. Hauser R, Yogev L, Greif M, Hirshenbein A, Botchan A, Gamzu R, et al. Sperm binding and ultrasound changes after operative repair of varicocele: correlation with fecundity. Andrologia. 1997;29(3):145–7. (PubMed PMID: 9197919).

139. Vigil P, Wohler C, Bustos-Obregon E, Comhaire F, Morales P. Assessment of sperm function in fertile and infertile men. Andrologia. 1994;26(2):55–60. (PubMed PMID: 8042770).

140. Fuse H, Akashi T, Fujishiro Y, Kazama T, Katayama T. Effect of varicocele on fertility potential: comparison between impregnating and nonimpregnating groups. Arch Androl. 1995;35(2):143–8. (PubMed PMID: 8579475).

141. Yagi K. Simple procedure for specific assay of lipid hydroperoxides in serum or plasma. Methods Mol Biol. 1998;108:107–10. (PubMed PMID: 9921520).

142. Aitken RJ, Baker MA, O'Bryan M. Shedding light on chemiluminescence: the application of chemiluminescence in diagnostic andrology. J Androl. 2004;25(4):455–65. (PubMed PMID: 15223833).

143. Agarwal A, Cocuzza M, Abdelrazik H, Sharma RK. Oxidative stress measurement in patients with male or female factor infertility. In: Popv I, Lewin G, editors. Handbook of chemiluminescent methods in oxidative stress assessment [Internet]. Kerala: Tranworld Research Network, Trivandrum; 2008. p. 195–218.

144. Nallella KP, Allamaneni SS, Pasqualotto FF, Sharma RK, Thomas AJ Jr., Agarwal A. Relationship of interleukin-6 with semen characteristics and oxidative stress in patients with varicocele. Urology. 2004;64(5):1010–3. (PubMed PMID: 15533496).

145. Sharma RK, Pasqualotto FF, Nelson DR, Thomas AJ Jr., Agarwal A. The reactive oxygen species-total antioxidant capacity score is a new measure of oxidative stress to predict male infertility. Hum Reprod. 1999;14(11):2801–7. (PubMed PMID: 10548626).

146. Pasqualotto FF, Sharma RK, Nelson DR, Thomas AJ, Agarwal A. Relationship between oxidative stress, semen characteristics, and clinical diagnosis in men undergoing infertility investigation. Fertil Steril. 2000;73(3):459–64. (PubMed PMID: 10688996).

147. Pasqualotto FF, Sharma RK, Kobayashi H, Nelson DR, Thomas AJ Jr., Agarwal A. Oxidative stress in normospermic men undergoing infertility evaluation. J Androl. 2001;22(2):316–22. (PubMed PMID: 11229806).

148. Wu Q, Xing J, Xue W, Sun J, Wang X, Jin X. Influence of polymorphism of glutathione S-transferase T1 on Chinese infertile patients with varicocele. Fertil Steril. 2009;91(3):960–2. (PubMed PMID: 18163994).

149. Sakamoto Y, Ishikawa T, Kondo Y, Yamaguchi K, Fujisawa M. The assessment of oxidative stress in infertile patients with varicocele. BJU Int. 2008;101(12):1547–52. (PubMed PMID: 18294306).

150. Mehraban D, Ansari M, Keyhan H, Sedighi Gilani M, Naderi G, Esfehani F. Comparison of nitric oxide concentration in seminal fluid between infertile patients with and without varicocele and normal fertile men. Urol J. 2005;2(2):106–10. (PubMed PMID: 17629881).

151. Xu Y, Xu QY, Yang BH, Zhu XM, Peng YF. [Relationship of nitric oxide and nitric oxide synthase with varicocele infertility]. Zhonghua Nan Ke Xue. 2008;14(5):414–7. (PubMed PMID: 18572859).

152. Abd-Elmoaty MA, Saleh R, Sharma R, Agarwal A. Increased levels of oxidants and reduced antioxidants in semen of infertile men with varicocele. Fertil Steril. 2010;94(4):1531–4. (PubMed PMID: 20117772).

153. Mostafa T, Anis T, El Nashar A, Imam H, Osman I. Seminal plasma reactive oxygen species-antioxidants relationship with varicocele grade. Andrologia. 2012;44(1):66–9. (PubMed PMID: 21651600).

154. Mazzilli F, Rossi T, Marchesini M, Ronconi C, Dondero F. Superoxide anion in human semen related to seminal parameters and clinical aspects. Fertil Steril. 1994;62(4):862–8. (PubMed PMID: 7926100).

155. Yesilli C, Mungan G, Seckiner I, Akduman B, Acikgoz S, Altan K, et al. Effect of varicocelectomy on sperm creatine kinase, HspA2 chaperone protein (creatine kinase-M type), LDH, LDH-X, and lipid peroxidation product levels in infertile men with varicocele. Urology. 2005;66(3):610–5. (PubMed PMID: 16140088).

156. Hurtado de Catalfo GE, Ranieri-Casilla A, Marra FA, de Alaniz MJ, Marra CA. Oxidative stress biomarkers and hormonal profile in human patients undergoing varicocelectomy. Int J Androl. 2007;30(6):519–30. (PubMed PMID: 17573856).

157. Akyol O, Ozbek E, Uz E, Kocak I. Malondialdehyde level and total superoxide dismutase activity in seminal fluid from patients with varicocele. Clin Exp Med. 2001;1(1):67–8. (PubMed PMID: 11467404).

158. Santoro G, Romeo C, Impellizzeri P, Ientile R, Cutroneo G, Trimarchi F, et al. Nitric oxide synthase patterns in normal and varicocele testis in adolescents. BJU Int. 2001;88(9):967–73. (PubMed PMID: 11851622).

159. Shiraishi K, Naito K. Nitric oxide produced in the testis is involved in dilatation of the internal spermatic vein that compromises spermatogenesis in infertile men with varicocele. BJU Int. 2007;99(5):1086–90. (PubMed PMID: 17346270).

160. Ishikawa T, Fujioka H, Ishimura T, Takenaka A, Fujisawa M. Increased testicular 8-hydroxy-2'-deoxyguanosine in patients with varicocele. BJU Int. 2007;100(4):863–6. (PubMed PMID: 17559562).

161. Shiraishi K, Takihara H, Matsuyama H. Elevated scrotal temperature, but not varicocele grade, reflects testicular oxidative stress-mediated apoptosis. World J Urol. 2010;28(3):359–64. (PubMed PMID: 19655149).

162. Koksal IT, Usta M, Orhan I, Abbasoglu S, Kadioglu A. Potential role of reactive oxygen species on testicular pathology associated with infertility. Asian J Androl. 2003;5(2):95–9. (PubMed PMID: 12778317. Epub 2003/06/05. eng).

163. Ozbek E, Ilbey YY, Simsek A, Cekmen M, Balbay MD. Preoperative and postoperative seminal nitric oxide levels in patients with infertile varicocele. Arch Ital Urol Androl. 2009;81(4):248–50. (PubMed PMID: 20608151).

164. Mostafa T, Anis TH, Ghazi S, El-Nashar AR, Imam H, Osman IA. Reactive oxygen species and antioxidants relationship in the internal spermatic vein blood of infertile men with varicocele. Asian J Androl. 2006;8(4):451–4. (PubMed PMID: 16763721).

165. Romeo C, Ientile R, Impellizzeri P, Turiaco N, Teletta M, Antonuccio P, et al. Preliminary report on nitric oxide-mediated oxidative damage in adolescent varicocele. Hum Reprod. 2003;18(1):26–9. (PubMed PMID: 12525436).

166. Turkyilmaz Z, Gulen S, Sonmez K, Karabulut R, Dincer S, Can Basaklar A, et al. Increased nitric oxide is accompanied by lipid oxidation in adolescent varicocele. Int J Androl. 2004;27(3):183–7. (PubMed PMID: 15139975).

167. Chen SS, Chang LS, Wei YH. Oxidative damage to proteins and decrease of antioxidant capacity in patients with varicocele. Free Radic Biol Med. 2001;30(11):1328–34. (PubMed PMID: 11368931).

168. Giulini S, Sblendorio V, Xella S, La Marca A, Palmieri B, Volpe A. Seminal plasma total antioxidant capacity and semen parameters in patients with varicocele. Reprod Biomed Online. 2009;18(5):617–21. (PubMed PMID: 19549438).

169. Mancini A, Milardi D, Bianchi A, Festa R, Silvestrini A, De Marinis L, et al. Increased total antioxidant capacity in seminal plasma of varicocele patients: a multivariate analysis. Arch Androl. 2007;53(1):37–42. (PubMed PMID: 17364464. Epub 2007/03/17. eng).

170. Agarwal A. Role of oxidative stress in in male infer tility and antioxidant supplementation. Business briefing: US kidney & urological disease [Internet]. 2005. 122–5 pp. December 2011. http://www.clevelandclinic.org/reproductiveresearchcenter/docs/agradoc174.pdf.

171. Kanter M, Aktas C, Erboga M. Heat stress decreases testicular germ cell proliferation and increases apoptosis in short term: an immunohistochemical and ultrastructural study. Toxicol Ind Health. 2013;29(2):99–113. (PubMed PMID: 22082826. Epub 2011/11/16. Eng).

172. Pigeolet E, Corbisier P, Houbion A, Lambert D, Michiels C, Raes M, et al. Glutathione peroxidase, superoxide dismutase, and catalase inactivation by peroxides and oxygen derived free radicals. Mech Ageing Dev. 1990;51(3):283–97. (PubMed PMID: 2308398. Epub 1990/02/15. eng).

173. Zini A, Schlegel PN. Cu/Zn superoxide dismutase, catalase and glutathione peroxidase mRNA expression in the rat testis after surgical cryptorchidism and efferent duct ligation. J Urol. 1997;158(2):659–63. (PubMed PMID: 9224387. Epub 1997/08/01. eng).

174. Peltola V, Huhtaniemi I, Ahotupa M. Abdominal position of the rat testis is associated with high level of lipid peroxidation. Biol Reprod. 1995;53(5):1146–50. (PubMed PMID: 8527519).

175. Gulyaeva NV, Obidin AB, Marinov BS. Modulation of superoxide dismutase by electron donors and acceptors. FEBS Lett. 1987;211(2):211–4. (PubMed PMID: 2433158. Epub 1987/01/26. eng).

176. Peltola V, Huhtaniemi I, Ahotupa M. Antioxidant enzyme activity in the maturing rat testis. J Androl. 1992;13(5):450–5. (PubMed PMID: 1429221. Epub 1992/09/01. eng).

177. Wang YJ, Zhang RQ, Lin YJ, Zhang RG, Zhang WL. Relationship between varicocele and sperm DNA damage and the effect of varicocele repair: a meta-analysis. Reprod Biomed Online. 2012;25(3):307–14. (PubMed PMID: 22809864).

178. Dubin L, Amelar RD. Etiologic factors in 1294 consecutive cases of male infertility. Fertil Steril. 1971;22(8):469–74. (PubMed PMID: 4398669).

179. Agarwal A, Deepinder F, Cocuzza M, Agarwal R, Short RA, Sabanegh E, et al. Efficacy of varicocelectomy in improving semen parameters: new meta-analytical approach. Urology. 2007;70(3):532–8. (PubMed PMID: 17905111).

180. Evers JL, Collins JA, Vandekerckhove P. Surgery or embolisation for varicocele in subfertile men. Cochrane Database Syst Rev. 2001 (1):CD000479. (PubMed PMID: 11279693).

181. Ficarra V, Cerruto MA, Liguori G, Mazzoni G, Minucci S, Tracia A, et al. Treatment of varicocele in subfertile men: the Cochrane Review–a contrary opinion. Eur Urol. 2006;49(2):258–63. (PubMed PMID: 16426727).

182. Marmar JL, Agarwal A, Prabakaran S, Agarwal R, Short RA, Benoff S, et al. Reassessing the value of varicocelectomy as a treatment for male subfertility with a new meta-analysis. Fertil Steril. 2007;88(3):639–48. (PubMed PMID: 17434508).

183. Mancini A, Conte G, Milardi D, De Marinis L, Littarru GP. Relationship between sperm cell ubiquinone and seminal parameters in subjects with and without varicocele. Andrologia. 1998;30(1):1–4. (PubMed PMID: 9567163).

184. Gat Y, Bachar GN, Zukerman Z, Belenky A, Gorenish M. Physical examination may miss the diagnosis of bilateral varicocele: a comparative study of 4 diagnostic modalities. J Urol. 2004;172(4 Pt 1):1414–7. (PubMed PMID: 15371858).

185. Dubin L, Amelar RD. Varicocele size and results of varicocelectomy in selected subfertile men with varicocele. Fertil Steril. 1970;21(8):606–9. (PubMed PMID: 5433164).

186. Stahl P, Schlegel PN. Standardization and documentation of varicocele evaluation. Curr Opin Urol. 2011;21(6):500–5. (PubMed PMID: 21926627).

187. Liguori G, Trombetta C, Garaffa G, Bucci S, Gattuccio I, Salame L, et al. Color Doppler ultrasound investigation of varicocele. World J Urol. 2004;22(5):378–81. (PubMed PMID: 15322805).

188. Chiou RK, Anderson JC, Wobig RK, Rosinsky DE, Matamoros A Jr., Chen WS, et al. Color Doppler ultrasound criteria to diagnose varicoceles: correlation of a new scoring system with physical examination. Urology. 1997;50(6):953–6. (PubMed PMID: 9426729).

189. Pilatz A, Altinkilic B, Kohler E, Marconi M, Weidner W. Color Doppler ultrasound imaging in varicoceles: is the venous diameter sufficient for predicting clinical and subclinical varicocele? World J Urol. 2011;29(5):645–50. (PubMed PMID: 21607575).

190. Sarteschi LM, Paoli R, Bianchini M, Menchini Fabris GF Lo studio del varicocele con ecocolor Doppler. G Ital Ultrasonologia. 1993;4:43–9.

191. Kondoh N, Meguro N, Matsumiya K, Namiki M, Kiyohara H, Okuyama A. Significance of subclinical varicocele detected by scrotal sonography in male infertility: a preliminary report. J Urol. 1993;150(4):1158–60. (PubMed PMID: 8371378).

192. Ahlberg NE, Bartley O, Chidekel N, Fritjofsson A. Phlebography in varicocele scroti. Acta Radiol Diagn (Stockh). 1966;4(5):517–28. (PubMed PMID: 5920098).

193. Lindholmer C, Thulin L, Eliasson R. Concentrations of cortisol and renin in the internal spermatic vein of men with varicocele. Andrologie. 1973;5(1):21–2. (PubMed PMID: 4764202).

194. Narayan P, Amplatz K, Gonazlez R. Varicocele and male subfertility. Fertil Steril. 1981;36(1):92–7. (PubMed PMID: 7250412).

195. Nadel SN, Hutchins GM, Albertsen PC, White RI Jr. Valves of the internal spermatic vein: potential for misdiagnosis of varicocele by venography. Fertil Steril. 1984;41(3):479–81. (PubMed PMID: 6698242).

196. Rosenbaltt M, Dickey K. Varicocele and female infertility. In: Bakal CW, Silberzweig JE, Cynamon J, editors. Vascular and interventional radiology: principles and practice. New York: Thieme Medical Publisher; 2002. p. 317.

197. Marsman JW. Clinical versus subclinical varicocele: venographic findings and improvement of fertility after embolization. Radiology. 1985;155(3):635–8. (PubMed PMID: 4001363).

198. Sigmund G, Bahren W, Gall H, Lenz M, Thon W. Idiopathic varicoceles: feasibility of percutaneous sclerotherapy. Radiology. 1987;164(1):161–8. (PubMed PMID: 3588899).

199. Lawson R. Thermography; a new tool in the investigation of breast lesions. Can Serv Med J. 1957;8(8):517–24. (PubMed PMID: 13460932).

200. Mieusset R, Bujan L. Testicular heating and its possible contributions to male infertility: a review. Int J Androl. 1995;18(4):169–84. (PubMed PMID: 7591190).

201. Nogueira FE, Medeiros F, Barroso LV, Miranda EP, de Castro JD, Mota Filho FH. Infrared digital telethermography: a new method for early detection of varicocele. Fertil Steril. 2009;92(1):361–2. (PubMed PMID: 19100536).

202. Gat Y, Bachar GN, Zukerman Z, Belenky A, Gornish M. Varicocele: a bilateral disease. Fertil Steril. 2004;81(2):424–9. (PubMed PMID: 14967384).

203. Yamamoto M, Hibi H, Hirata Y, Miyake K, Ishigaki T. Effect of varicocelectomy on sperm parameters and pregnancy rate in patients with subclinical varicocele: a randomized prospective controlled study. J Urol. 1996;155(5):1636–8. (PubMed PMID: 8627841).

204. Watanabe Y. Scrotal imaging. Curr Opin Urol. 2002;12(2):149–53. (PubMed PMID: 11859263).

205. Hirsh AV, Kellett MJ, Robertson G, Pryor JP. Doppler flow studies, venography and thermography in the evaluation of varicoceles of fertile and subfertile men. Br J Urol. 1980;52(6):560–5. (PubMed PMID: 7459590).

206. Kormano M, Kahanpaa K, Svinhufvud U, Tahti E. Thermography of varicocele. Fertil Steril. 1970;21(7):558–64. (PubMed PMID: 5433669).

207. Pochaczevsky R, Lee WJ, Mallett E. Management of male infertility: roles of contact thermography, spermatic venography, and embolization. AJR Am J Roentgenol. 1986;147(1):97–102. (PubMed PMID: 3487239).

208. Mieusset R, Bujan L, Mondinat C, Mansat A, Pontonnier F, Grandjean H. Association of scrotal hyperthermia with impaired spermatogenesis in infertile men. Fertil Steril. 1987;48(6):1006–11. (PubMed PMID: 3678498).

209. Abbasi M, Alizadeh R, Abolhassani F, Amidi F, Hassanzadeh G, Ejtemaei Mehr S, et al. Aminoguanidine improves epididymal sperm parameters in varicocelized rats. Urol Int. 2011;86(3):302–6. (PubMed PMID: 21088382. Epub 2010/11/23. eng).

210. Abbasi M, Alizadeh R, Abolhassani F, Amidi F, Ragerdi KI, Fazelipour S, et al. Effect of aminoguanidine in sperm DNA fragmentation in varicocelized rats: role of nitric oxide. Reprod Sci. 2011;18(6):545–50. (PubMed PMID: 21285452. Epub 2011/02/03. eng).

211. Cam K, Simsek F, Yuksel M, Turkeri L, Haklar G, Yalcin S, et al. The role of reactive oxygen species and apoptosis in the pathogenesis of varicocele in a rat model and efficiency of vitamin E treatment. Int J Androl. 2004;27(4):228–33. (PubMed PMID: 15271202).

212. Oliva A, Dotta A, Multigner L. Pentoxifylline and antioxidants improve sperm quality in male patients with varicocele. Fertil Steril. 2009;91(4 Suppl):1536–9. (PubMed PMID: 18990381).

213. Cavallini G, Ferraretti AP, Gianaroli L, Biagiotti G, Vitali G. Cinnoxicam and L-carnitine/acetyl-L-carnitine treatment for idiopathic and varicocele-associated oligoasthenospermia. J Androl. 2004;25(5):761–70; discussion 71–2. (PubMed PMID: 15292108).

214. Cavallini G, Biagiotti G, Ferraretti AP, Gianaroli L, Vitali G. Medical therapy of oligoasthenospermia associated with left varicocele. BJU Int. 2003;91(6):513–8. (PubMed PMID: 12656905).

215. Qu XW, Shan ZJ, Han QH, Hu JT, Zhang PH, Zhang SW. [Effects of Qiangjing Capsule on the oxidative and antioxidative system in the epididymis of varicocele rats]. Zhonghua Nan Ke Xue. 2011;17(11):1039–42. (PubMed PMID: 22141278. Epub 2011/12/07. chi).

216. Zampieri N, Pellegrino M, Ottolenghi A, Camoglio FS. Effects of bioflavonoids in the management of subclinical varicocele. Pediatr Surg Int. 2010;26(5):505–8. (PubMed PMID: 20162420).

217. Kilic S, Gunes A, Ipek D, Dusak A, Gunes G, Balbay MD, et al. Effects of micronised purified flavonoid fraction on pain, spermiogram and scrotal color Doppler parameters in patients with painful varicocele. Urol Int. 2005;74(2):173–9. (PubMed PMID: 15756071).

218. Paradiso Galatioto G, Gravina GL, Angelozzi G, Sacchetti A, Innominato PF, Pace G, et al. May antioxidant therapy improve sperm parameters of men with persistent oligospermia after retrograde embolization for varicocele? World J Urol. 2008;26(1):97–102. (PubMed PMID: 17982752).

219. Takihara H, Cosentino MJ, Cockett AT. Zinc sulfate therapy for infertile male with or without varicocelectomy. Urology. 1987;29(6):638–41. (PubMed PMID: 3576896).

220. Yan LF, Jiang MF, Shao RY. [Clinical observation on effect of jingling oral liquid in treating infertile patients with varicocele after varicocelectomy]. Zhongguo Zhong Xi Yi Jie He Za Zhi. 2004;24(3):220–2. (PubMed PMID: 15074089).

221. Esteves SC, Agarwal A. Novel concepts in male infertility. Int Braz J Urol. 2011;37(1):5–15. (PubMed PMID: 21385475. Epub 2011/03/10. eng).

222. Geatti O, Gasparini D, Shapiro B. A comparison of scintigraphy, thermography, ultrasound and phlebography in grading of clinical varicocele. J Nucl Med. 1991;32(11):2092–7. (PubMed PMID: 1941143).

223. World Health Organization (WHO). WHO laboratory manual for the examination and processing of human semen. 5th ed. Geneva: World Health Organization Press; 2010.

224. Steckel J, Dicker AP, Goldstein M. Relationship between varicocele size and response to varicocelectomy. J Urol. 1993;149:769–71.

225. Marks JL, McMahon R, Lipshultz LI. Predictive parameters of successful varicocele repair. J Urol. 1986;136(3):609–12. (PubMed PMID: 3090279).

226. Yoshida K, Kitahara S, Chiba K, Horiuchi S, Horimi H, Sumi S, et al. Predictive indicators of successful varicocele repair in men with infertility. Int J Fertil Womens Med. 2000;45(4):279–84. (PubMed PMID: 10997484).

227. Cayan S, Lee D, Black LD, Reijo Pera RA, Turek PJ. Response to varicocelectomy in oligospermic men with and without defined genetic infertility. Urology. 2001;57(3):530–5. (PubMed PMID: 11248633).

228. Pryor JL, Kent-First M, Muallem A, Van Bergen AH, Nolten WE, Meisner L, et al. Microdeletions in the Y chromosome of infertile men. N Engl J Med. 1997;336(8):534–9. (PubMed PMID: 9023089).

229. Kondo Y, Ishikawa T, Yamaguchi K, Fujisawa M. Predictors of improved seminal characteristics by varicocele repair. Andrologia. 2009;41(1):20–3. (PubMed PMID: 19143725).

230. Esteves SC, Glina S. Recovery of spermatogenesis after microsurgical subinguinal varicocele repair in azoospermic men based on testicular histology. Int Braz J Urol. 2005;31(6):541–8. (PubMed PMID: 16386122).

231. Weedin JW, Khera M, Lipshultz LI. Varicocele repair in patients with nonobstructive azoospermia: a meta-analysis. J Urol. 2010;183(6):2309–15. (PubMed PMID: 20400156).

232. Esteves S. Varicocele. In: Parekattil SJ, Agarwal A, editors. Male infertility: contemporary clinical approaches, andrology, ART & antioxidants. 1st ed ed. New York: Springer; 2012. p. 247–59.

233. Cayan S, Shavakhabov S, Kadioglu A. Treatment of palpable varicocele in infertile men: a meta-analysis to define the best technique. J Androl. 2009;30(1):33–40. (PubMed PMID: 18772487).

234. Sautter T, Sulser T, Suter S, Gretener H, Hauri D. Treatment of varicocele: a prospective randomized comparison of laparoscopy versus antegrade sclerotherapy. Eur Urol. 2002;41(4):398–400. (PubMed PMID: 12074810).

235. Al-Kandari AM, Shabaan H, Ibrahim HM, Elshebiny YH, Shokeir AA. Comparison of outcomes of different varicocelectomy techniques: open inguinal, laparoscopic, and subinguinal microscopic varicocelectomy: a randomized clinical trial. Urology. 2007;69(3):417–20. (PubMed PMID: 17382134).

236. Hopps CV, Lemer ML, Schlegel PN, Goldstein M. Intraoperative varicocele anatomy: a microscopic study of the inguinal versus subinguinal approach. J Urol. 2003;170(6 Pt 1):2366–70. (PubMed PMID: 14634418).

237. Esteves SC, Miyaoka R, Agarwal A. Surgical treatment of male infertility in the era of intracytoplasmic sperm injection—new insights. Clinics. 2011;66(8):1463–78. (PubMed PMID: 21915501. Pubmed Central PMCID: 3161229).

238. Esteves SC, Oliveira FV, Bertolla RP. Clinical outcome of intracytoplasmic sperm injection in infertile men with treated and untreated clinical varicocele. J Urol. 2010;184(4):1442–6. (PubMed PMID: 20727535).

239. Cocuzza M, Pagani R, Coelho R, Srougi M, Hallak J. The systematic use of intraoperative vascular Doppler ultrasound during microsurgical subinguinal varicocelectomy improves precise identification and preservation of testicular blood supply. Fertil Steril. 2010;93(7):2396–9. (PubMed PMID: 19268931).

240. Soylemez H, Kilic S, Atar M, Penbegul N, Sancaktutar AA, Bozkurt Y. Effects of micronised purified flavonoid fraction on pain, semen analysis and scrotal color Doppler parameters in patients with painful varicocele; results of a randomized placebo-controlled study. Int Urol Nephrol. 2012;44(2):401–8. (PubMed PMID: 21805085).

241. Nieschlag E, Hertle L, Fischedick A, Abshagen K, Behre HM. Update on treatment of varicocele: counselling as effective as occlusion of the vena spermatica. Hum Reprod. 1998;13(8):2147–50. (PubMed PMID: 9756286).

242. Evers JL, Collins JA. Surgery or embolisation for varicocele in subfertile men. Cochrane Database Syst Rev. 2004 (3):CD000479. (PubMed PMID: 15266431).
243. Practice Committee of the American Society for Reproductive M. Report on varicocele and infertility. Fertil Steril. 2006;86(5 Suppl 1):S93–5. (PubMed PMID: 17055852).
244. Unal D, Yeni E, Verit A, Karatas OF. Clomiphene citrate versus varicocelectomy in treatment of subclinical varicocele: a prospective randomized study. Int J Urol. 2001;8(5):227–30. (PubMed PMID: 11328423).
245. Zheng YQ, Gao X, Li ZJ, Yu YL, Zhang ZG, Li W. Efficacy of bilateral and left varicocelectomy in infertile men with left clinical and right subclinical varicoceles: a comparative study. Urology. 2009;73(6):1236–40. (PubMed PMID: 19371942).
246. Elbendary MA, Elbadry AM. Right subclinical varicocele: how to manage in infertile patients with clinical left varicocele? Fertil Steril. 2009;92(6):2050–3. (PubMed PMID: 19615680).
247. Amelar RD, Dubin L. Right varicocelectomy in selected infertile patients who have failed to improve after previous left varicocelectomy. Fertil Steril. 1987;47(5):833–7. (PubMed PMID: 3569559).
248. Projeto Diretrizes da Associac¸ao Me´dica. Brasileira: Varicocele. http://www.projetodiretrizes.org.br/8volume/40-Varicocele.pdf. (2011)
249. Guidelines on male infertility. 2010.
250. Pasqualotto FF, Lucon AM, de Goes PM, Sobreiro BP, Hallak J, Pasqualotto EB, et al. Is it worthwhile to operate on subclinical right varicocele in patients with grade II–III varicocele in the left testicle? J Assist Reprod Genet. 2005;22(5):227–31. (PubMed PMID: 16047585. Pubmed Central PMCID: 3455497).
251. Bong GW KH. The adolescent varicocele: to treat or not to treat. Urol Clin North Am. 2004;31:509–15.
252. Laven JS HL, Mali WP, te Velde ER, Wensing CJ, Eimers JM. Effects of varicocele treatment in adolescents: a randomized study. Fertil Steril. 1992;58:756–62.
253. Pinto KJ KR, Jarow JP. Varicocele related testicular atrophy and its predictive effect upon fertility. J Urol. 1994;152(2):788–90.
254. Okuyama A, Nakamura M, Namiki M, Takeyama M, Utsunomiya M, Fujioka H, et al. Surgical repair of varicocele at puberty: preventive treatment for fertility improvement. J Urol. 1988;139:562–4.
255. Mori MM, Bertolla RP, Fraietta R, Ortiz V, Cedenho AP. Does varicocele grade determine extent of alteration to spermatogenesis in adolescents? Fertil Steril. 2008;90(5):1769–73. (PubMed PMID: 18166185).
256. Esteves SC, Zini A, Aziz N, Alvarez JG, Sabanegh ES Jr., Agarwal A. Critical appraisal of World Health Organization's new reference values for human semen characteristics and effect on diagnosis and treatment of subfertile men. Urology. 2012;79(1):16–22. (PubMed PMID: 22070891).
257. Ding H, Tian J, Du W, et al. Open non-microsurgical, laparoscopic or open microsurgical varicocelectomy for male infertility: a meta-analysis of randomized controlled trials. BJU Int. 2012;110(10):1536–42.
258. Kass EJ, Belman A. Reversal of testicular growth by varicocele ligation. J Urol. 1987;137(3):475–6.
259. Okuyama A, Fujisue H, Matsui T, et al. Preoperative parameters related to the improvement of semen characteristics after surgical repair of varicocele in subfertile men. Eur Urol. 1988;14:442–6.
260. Decastro GJ SA, Poon SA, Laor L, Glassberg KI. Adolescent varicocelectomy-is the potential for catch-up growth related to age and/or Tanner stage?. J Urol. 2009;181:322–7.
261. Li F, Chiba K, Yamaguchi K, Okada K, Matsushita K, Ando M, et al. Effect of varicocelectomy on testicular volume in children and adolescents: a meta-analysis. Urology. 2012;79(6):1340–5. (PubMed PMID: 22516359).
262. Glassberg KI, Korets R. Update on the management of adolescent varicocele. F1000 Med Rep. 2010;2:25. (PubMed PMID: 20948860. Pubmed Central PMCID: 2948392).

263. Goldstein M, Gilbert BR, Dicker AP, Dwosh J, Gnecco C. Microsurgical inguinal varicocelectomy with delivery of the testis: an artery and lymphatic sparing technique. J Urol. 1992;148(6):1808–11. (PubMed PMID: 1433614).

264. Kocvara R, Dvoracek J, Sedlacek J, Dite Z, Novak K. Lymphatic sparing laparoscopic varicocelectomy: a microsurgical repair. J Urol. 2005;173(5):1751–4. (PubMed PMID: 15821575).

265. Marmar J, Benoff S. New scientific information related to varicoceles. J Urol. 2003;170(6 Pt 1):2371–3. (PubMed PMID: 14634419).

266. Cook DJ, Sackett DL, Spitzer WO. Methodologic guidelines for systematic reviews of randomized control trials in health care from the Potsdam Consultation on meta-analysis. J Clin Epidemiol. 1995;48(1):167–71. (PubMed PMID: 7853043).

267. Colpi GM, Carmignani L, Nerva F, Piediferro G, Castiglioni F, Grugnetti C, et al. Surgical treatment of varicocele by a subinguinal approach combined with antegrade intraoperative sclerotherapy of venous vessels. BJU Int. 2006;97(1):142–5. (PubMed PMID: 16336345).

268. Matkov TG, Zenni M, Sandlow J, Levine LA. Preoperative semen analysis as a predictor of seminal improvement following varicocelectomy. Fertil Steril. 2001;75(1):63–8. (PubMed PMID: 11163818).

269. Zini A, Boman J, Jarvi K, Baazeem A. Varicocelectomy for infertile couples with advanced paternal age. Urology. 2008;72(1):109–13. (PubMed PMID: 18384862).

270. Bozkurt Y, Soylemez H, Sancaktutar AA, Islamoglu Y, Kar A, Penbegul N, et al. Relationship between mean platelet volume and varicocele: a preliminary study. Urology. 2012;79(5):1048–51. (PubMed PMID: 22381251).

271. Rodriguez Pena M, Alescio L, Russell A, Lourenco da Cunha J, Alzu G, Bardoneschi E. Predictors of improved seminal parameters and fertility after varicocele repair in young adults. Andrologia. 2009;41(5):277–81. (PubMed PMID: 19737275).

272. Lacerda JI, Del Giudice PT, da Silva BF, Nichi M, Fariello RM, Fraietta R, et al. Adolescent varicocele: improved sperm function after varicocelectomy. Fertil Steril. 2011;95(3):994–9. (PubMed PMID: 21074153).

273. Esteves SC. Clinical management of infertile men with nonobstructive azoospermia. Asian J Androl. 2015;17(3):459–70. (PubMed PMID: 25677138).

274. Smit M, Romijn JC, Wildhagen MF, Veldhoven JL, Weber RF, Dohle GR. Decreased sperm DNA fragmentation after surgical varicocelectomy is associated with increased pregnancy rate. J Urol. 2013;189(1 Suppl):S146–50. (PubMed PMID: 23234621).

275. Kroese AC, de Lange NM, Collins J, Evers JL. Surgery or embolization for varicoceles in subfertile men. Cochrane Database Syst Rev. 2012;10:CD000479. (PubMed PMID: 23076888).

276. Inci K, Hascicek M, Kara O, Dikmen AV, Gurgan T, Ergen A. Sperm retrieval and intracytoplasmic sperm injection in men with nonobstructive azoospermia, and treated and untreated varicocele. J Urol. 2009;182(4):1500–5. (PubMed PMID: 19683732).

277. Freire GC. Surgery or embolization for varicoceles in subfertile men. Sao Paulo Med J. 2013;131(1):67. (PubMed PMID: 23538601).

278. Shindel AW, Yan Y, Naughton CK. Does the number and size of veins ligated at left-sided microsurgical subinguinal varicocelectomy affect semen analysis outcomes? Urology. 2007;69(6):1176–80. (PubMed PMID: 17572210).

279. Cocuzza M, Cocuzza MA, Bragais FM, Agarwal A. The role of varicocele repair in the new era of assisted reproductive technology. Clinics. 2008;63(3):395–404. (PubMed PMID: 18568252. Pubmed Central PMCID: 2664231).

280. Verit A. Re: Attenuation of oxidative stress after varicocelectomy in subfertile patients with varicocele: S. S. Chen, W. J. Huang, L. S. Chang and Y. H. Wei. J Urol 2008; 179:639–42. (J Urol. 2008 Sep;180(3):1190; author reply-1. (PubMed PMID: 18639896)).

281. Libman J, Jarvi K, Lo K, Zini A. Beneficial effect of microsurgical varicocelectomy is superior for men with bilateral versus unilateral repair. J Urol. 2006;176(6 Pt 1):2602–5; discussion 5. (PubMed PMID: 17085170).

282. Jeng SY, Wu SM, Lee JD. Cadmium accumulation and metallothionein overexpression in internal spermatic vein of patients with varicocele. Urology. 2009;73(6):1231–5. (PubMed PMID: 19362335).

283. Chen SS, Huang WJ, Chang LS, Wei YH. Attenuation of oxidative stress after varicocelectomy in subfertile patients with varicocele. J Urol. 2008;179(2):639–42. (PubMed PMID: 18082213).

284. Baazeem A, Belzile E, Ciampi A, Dohle G, Jarvi K, Salonia A, et al. Varicocele and male factor infertility treatment: a new meta-analysis and review of the role of varicocele repair. Eur Urol. 2011;60(4):796–808. (PubMed PMID: 21733620).

285. Jarow JP, Espeland MA, Lipshultz LI. Evaluation of the azoospermic patient. J Urol. 1989;142(1):62–5. (PubMed PMID: 2499695).

286. Pagani R, Brugh VM, 3rd, Lamb DJ. Y chromosome genes and male infertility. Urol Clin North Am. 2002;29(4):745–53. (PubMed PMID: 12516749).

287. Esteves SC, Miyaoka R, Agarwal A. Sperm retrieval techniques for assisted reproduction. Int Braz J Urol. 2011;37(5):570–83. (PubMed PMID: 22099268).

288. Hamada AJ, Esteves SC, Agarwal A. A comprehensive review of genetics and genetic testing in azoospermia. Clinics. 2013;68 Suppl 1:39–60. (PubMed PMID: 23503954. Pubmed Central PMCID: 3583155).

289. Krausz C, Hoefsloot L, Simoni M, Tuttelmann F, European Academy of Andrology, European Molecular Genetics Quality Network. EAA/EMQN best practice guidelines for molecular diagnosis of Y-chromosomal microdeletions: state-of-the-art 2013. Andrology. 2014;2(1):5–19. (PubMed PMID: 24357628. Pubmed Central PMCID: 4065365).

290. Pasqualotto FF, Sobreiro BP, Hallak J, Pasqualotto EB, Lucon AM. Induction of spermatogenesis in azoospermic men after varicocelectomy repair: an update. Fertil Steril. 2006;85(3):635–9. (PubMed PMID: 16500331).

291. Elzanaty S. Varicocele repair in non-obstructive azoospermic men: diagnostic value of testicular biopsy—a meta-analysis. Scand J Urol. 2014;48(6):494–8. (PubMed PMID: 25001949).

292. Aboulghar MA, Mansour RT, Serour GI, Fahmy I, Kamal A, Tawab NA, et al. Fertilization and pregnancy rates after intracytoplasmic sperm injection using ejaculate semen and surgically retrieved sperm. Fertil Steril. 1997;68(1):108–11. (PubMed PMID: 9207593).

293. Schlegel PN, Kaufmann J. Role of varicocelectomy in men with nonobstructive azoospermia. Fertil Steril. 2004;81(6):1585–8. (PubMed PMID: 15193481).

294. Haydardedeoglu B, Turunc T, Kilicdag EB, Gul U, Bagis T. The effect of prior varicocelectomy in patients with nonobstructive azoospermia on intracytoplasmic sperm injection outcomes: a retrospective pilot study. Urology. 2010;75(1):83–6. (PubMed PMID: 19913887).

295. Penson DF, Paltiel A, Krumholz HM, Palter S. The cost-effectiveness of treatment for varicocele related infertility. J Urol. 2002;168:2490–4.

296. Schlegel PN, Goldstein M. Alternate indications for varicocele repair: nonobstructive azoospermia, pain, androgen deficiency and progressive testicular dysfunction. Fertil Steril. 2011;96:1288–93.

297. Meng MV, Greene K, Turek PJ. Surgery or assisted reproduction? A decision analysis of treatment costs in male infertility. J Urol. 2005;174:1926–31.

298. Kim JH. Surgical managements versus artificial reproductive technology in male infertility: cost effectiveness in Korea. Clin Exp Reprod Med. 2013;40:30–5.

299. Jarow J, Sigman M, Kolettis PN, Lipshultz L, McClure RD, Nangia AK et al. The optimal evaluation of the infertile male: best practice statement. 2010 [cited 2015 2/27/2015]. https://www.auanet.org/education/guidelines/male-infertility-d.cfm.

300. Practice Committee of the American Society for Reproductive Medicine, Society for Male Reproduction and Urology. Report on varicocele and infertility: a committee opinion. Fertil Steril. 2014;102(6):1556–60. (PubMed PMID: 25458620).

301. Jungwirth A, Diemer T, Dohle GR, Giwercman A, Kopa Z KC, Tournaye H. EAU Guidelines of male infertility 2013 [cited 2015 2/20/2015]. http://uroweb.org/guideline/male-infertility/.

302. Tekgul S, Dogan H, Erdem E, Hoebeke P, Kocvara R, Nijman JM, Radmayr C, Silay MS, Stein R, Undre S. EAU Guidelines on paediatric urology. 2015. http://www.uroweb.org/guideline/paediatric-urology/.
303. Graham R, Mancher M, Wolman DM, Greenfield S, Steinberg E. Institute of Medicine. Clinical practice guidelines we can trust. Washington (DC): National Academies Press; 2011. http://www.iom.edu/Reports/2011/Clinical-Practice-Guidelines-We-Can-Trust/Standards.aspx].
304. Trost LW, Nehra A. Guideline-based management of male infertility: Why do we need it? Indian J Urol. 2011;27(1):49–57. (PubMed PMID: 21716890. Pubmed Central PMCID: 3114588).
305. Aragona F, Ragazzi R, Pozzan GB, et al. Correlation of testicular volume, histology and LHRH test in adolescents with idiopathic varicocele. Eur Urol 1994;26(1):61–6.
306. Paduch DA, Niedzielski J. Repair versus observation in adolescent varicocele: a prospective study. J Urol. 1997;158:1128–32.
307. Yamamoto M, Katsuno S, Yokoi K, Hibi H, Miyake K. The effect of varicocelectomy on testicular volume in infertile patients with varicoceles. Nagoya J Med Sci. 1995;58(1–2):47–50. (PubMed PMID: 7659147).
308. Sigman M, Jarow JP. Ipsilateral testicular hypotrophy is associated with decreased sperm counts in infertile men with varicoceles. J Urol. 1997;158:605–7.
309. Abdel-Meguid T, Al-Sayyad A, Tayib A, et al. Does varicocele repair improve male infertility? An evidence-based perspective from a randomized, controlled trial. Eur Urol. 2011 59(3):455–61.
310. Chen JJ, Ahn H, Junewick J, et al. Is the comparison of a left varicocele testis to its contralateral normal testis sufficient in determining its well-being? Urology 2011;78(5):1167–72.